PICTURE BOOK OF
Horses

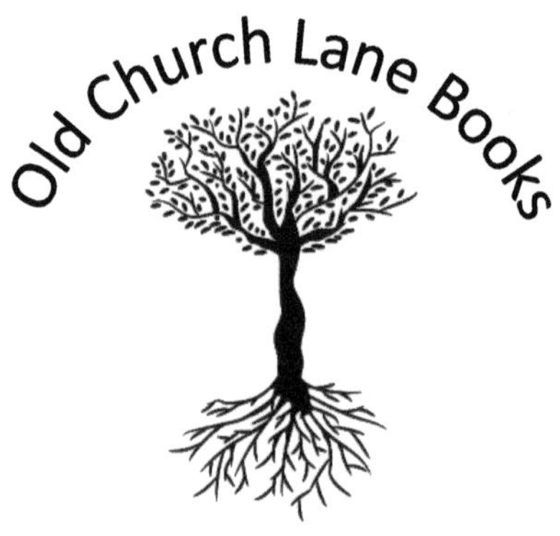

Old Church Lane Books

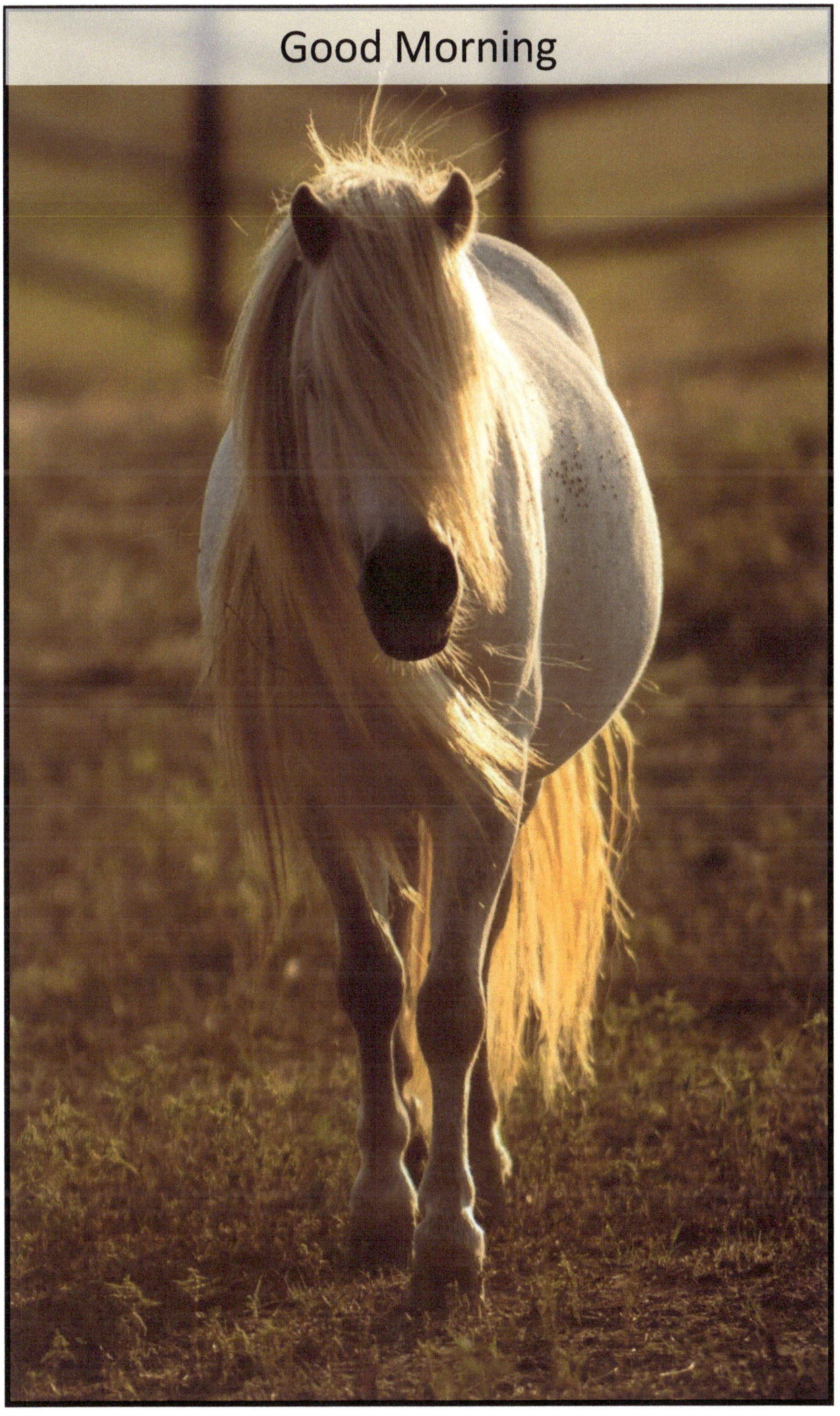

Good Morning

It Looks Like Twins

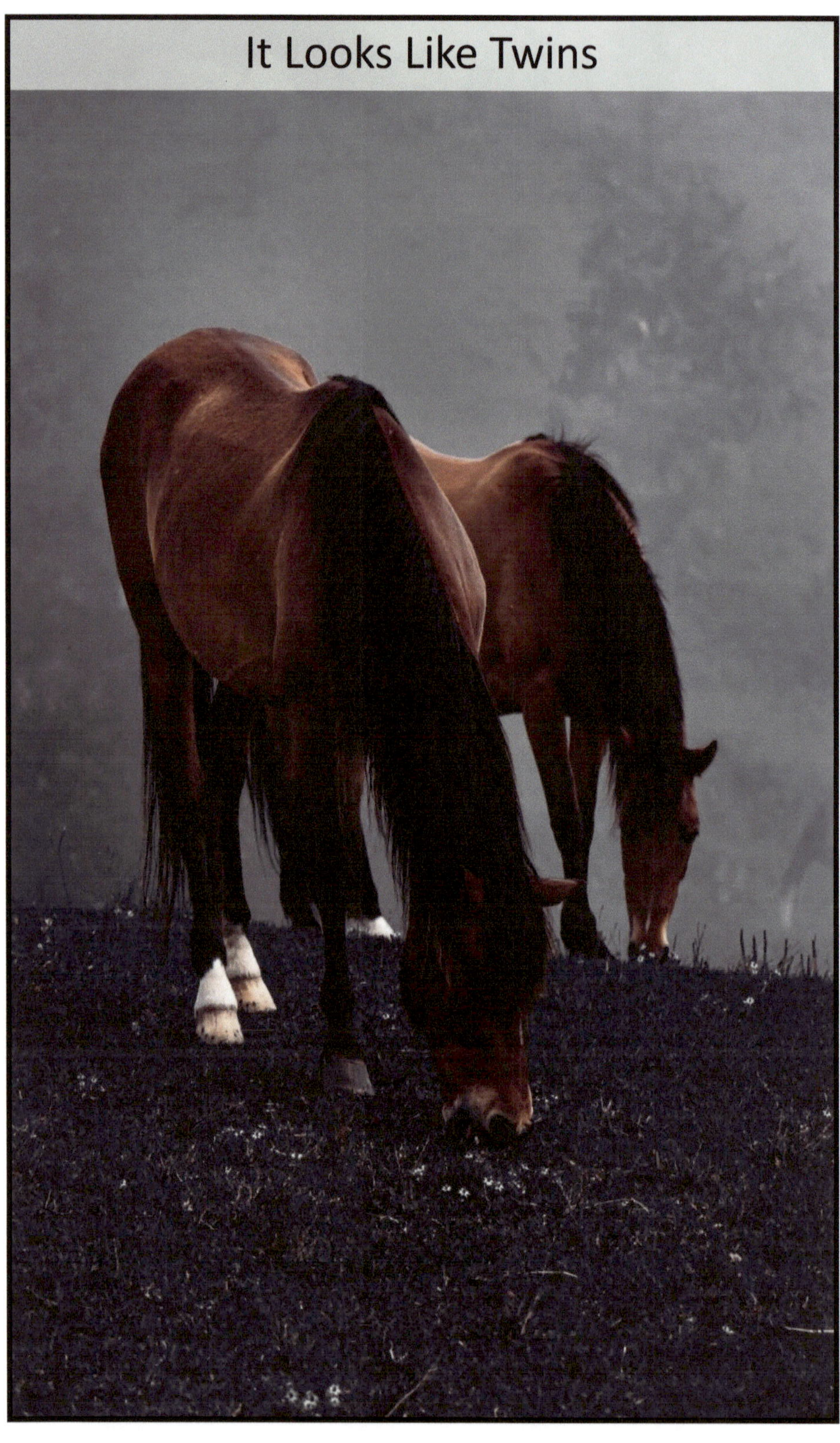

Hello Beautiful

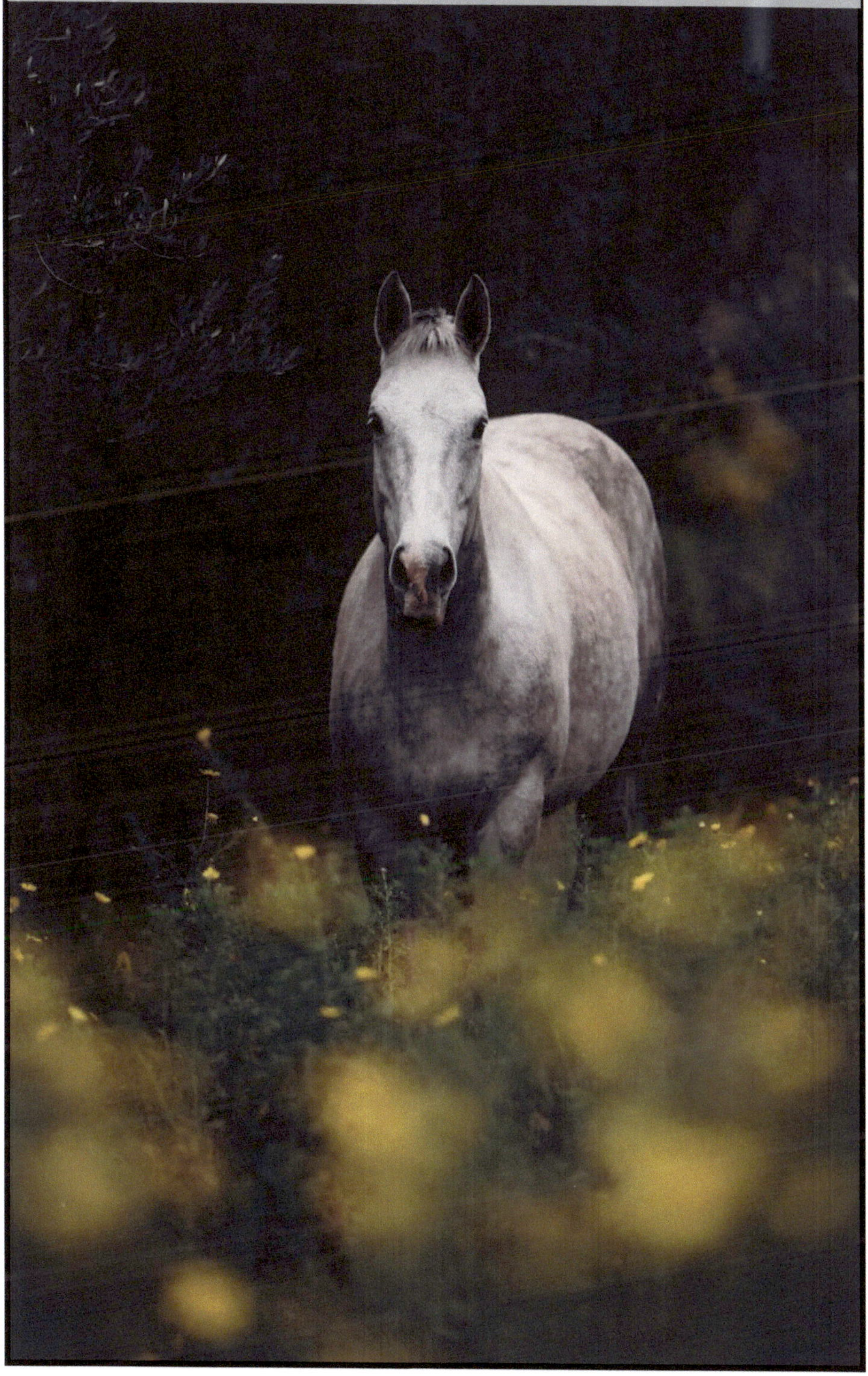

New Life

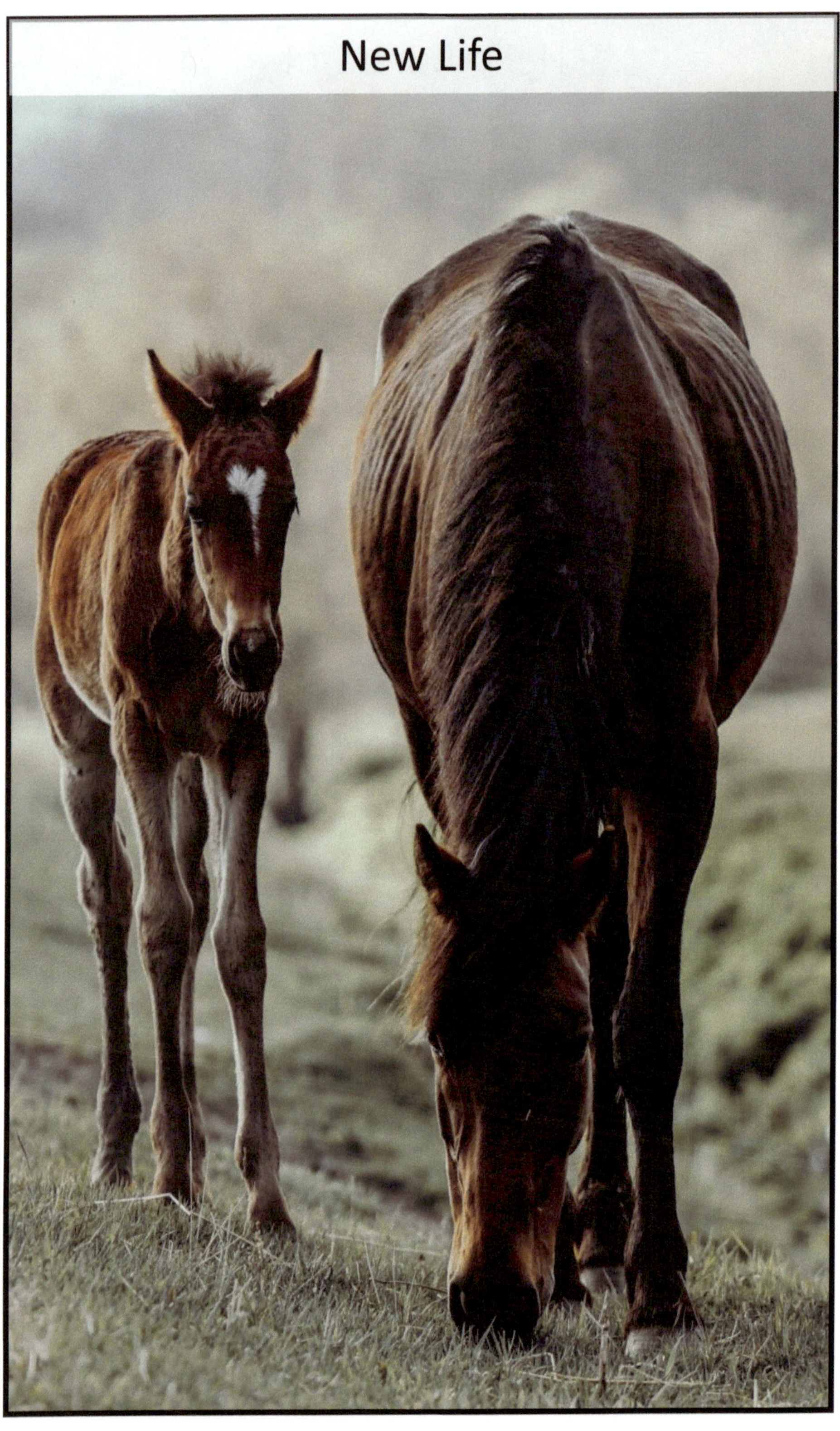

Please Let Me Out

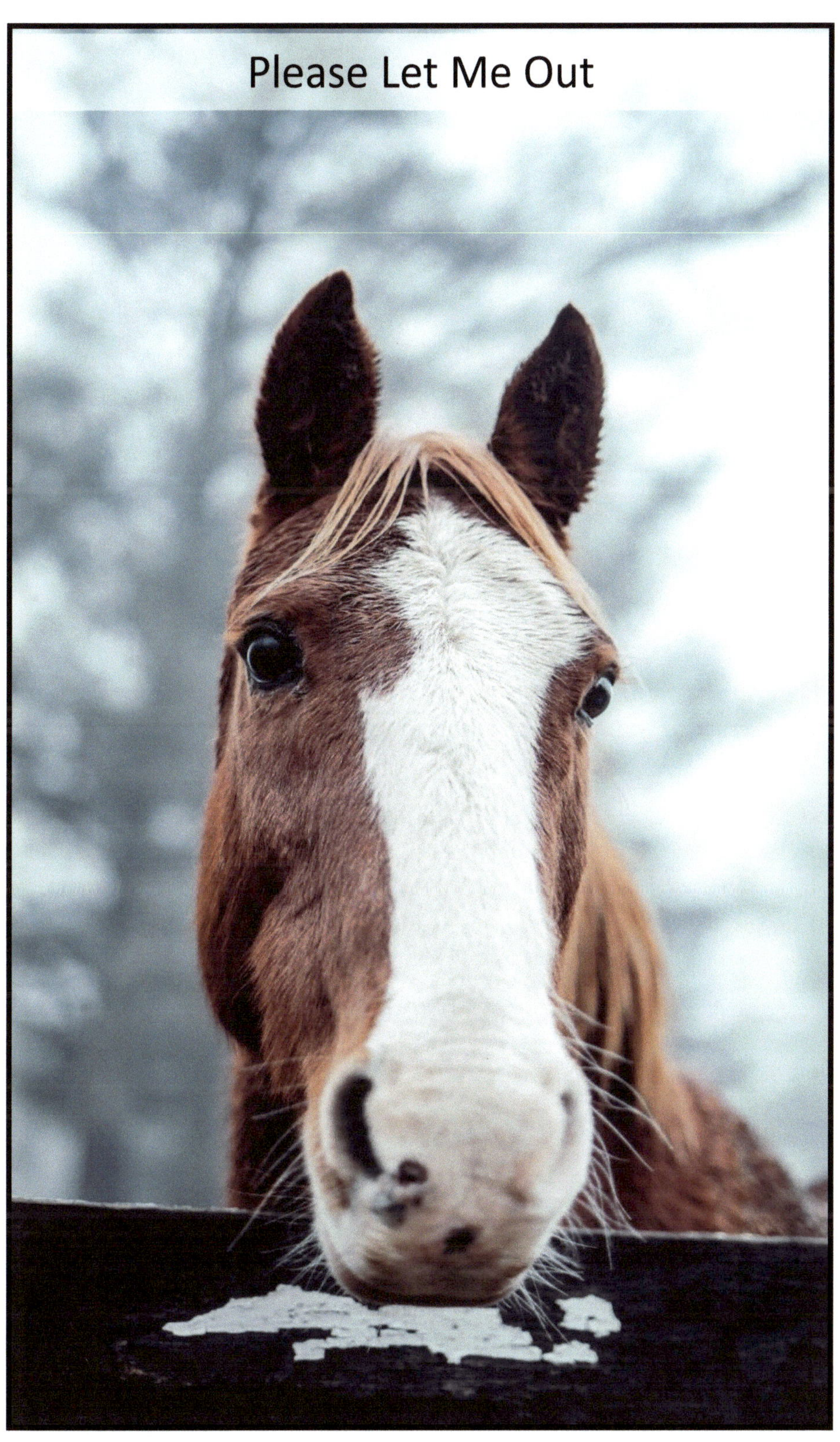

Brand New Day

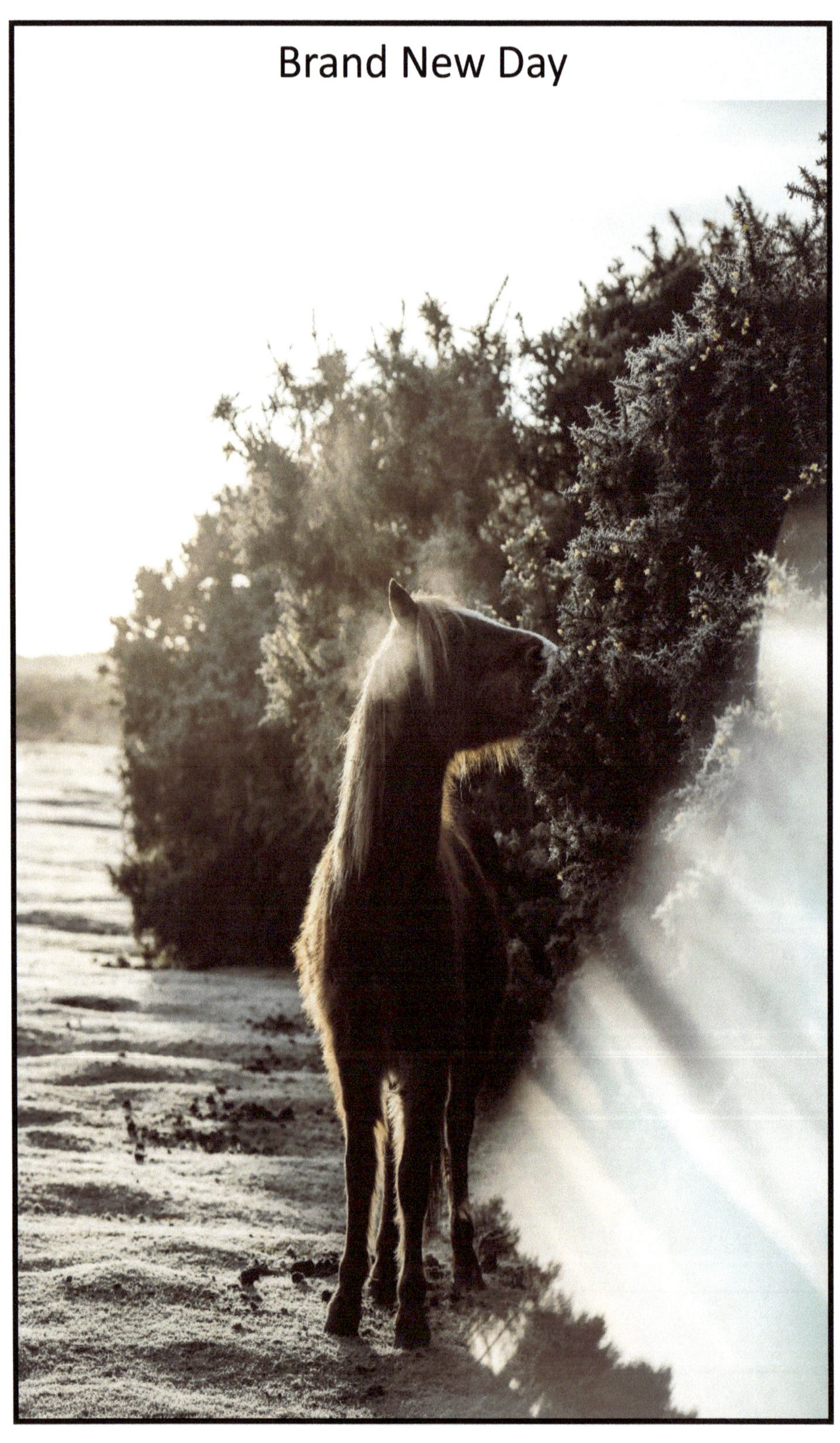

Breath Of Fresh Air

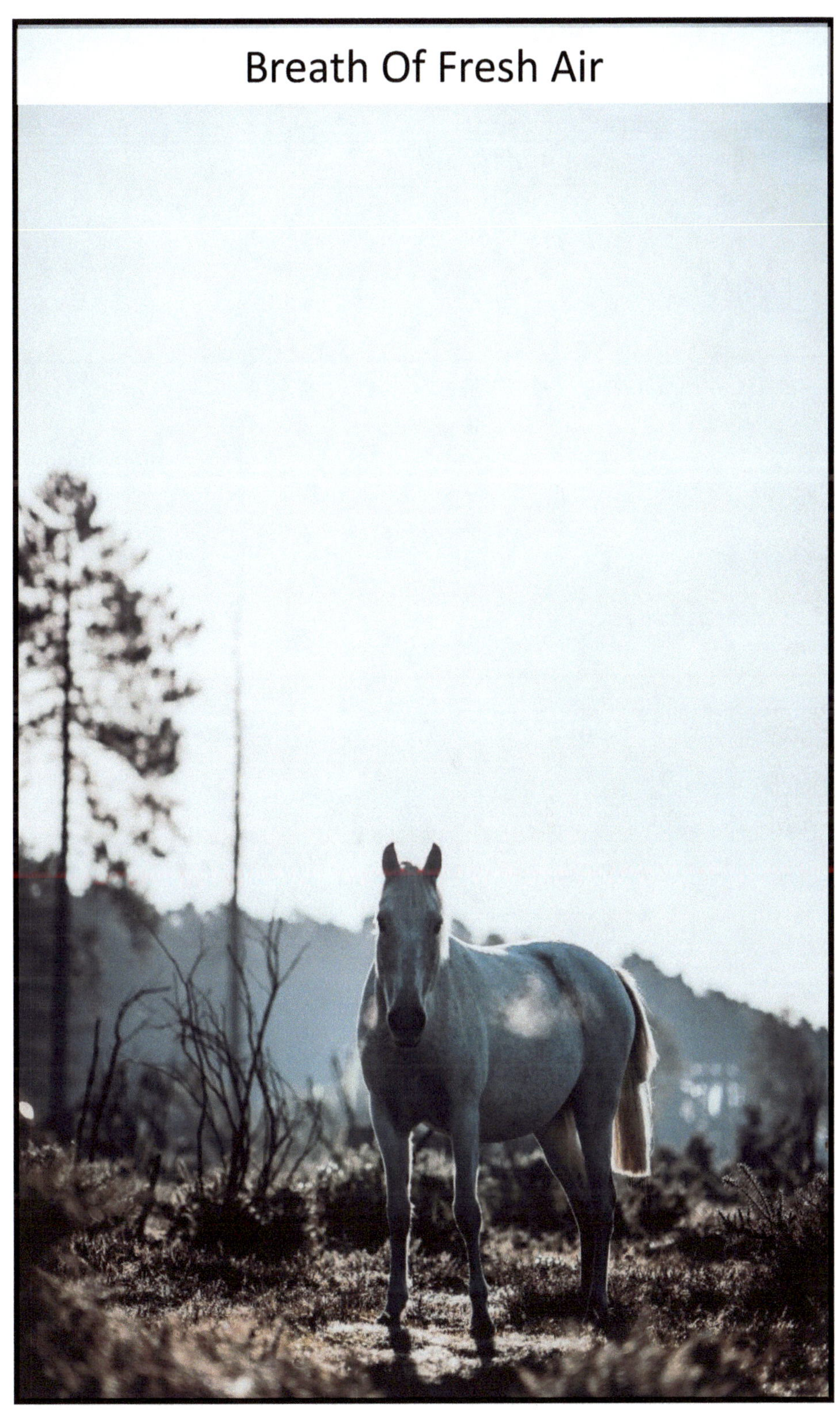

This IS My Happy Face

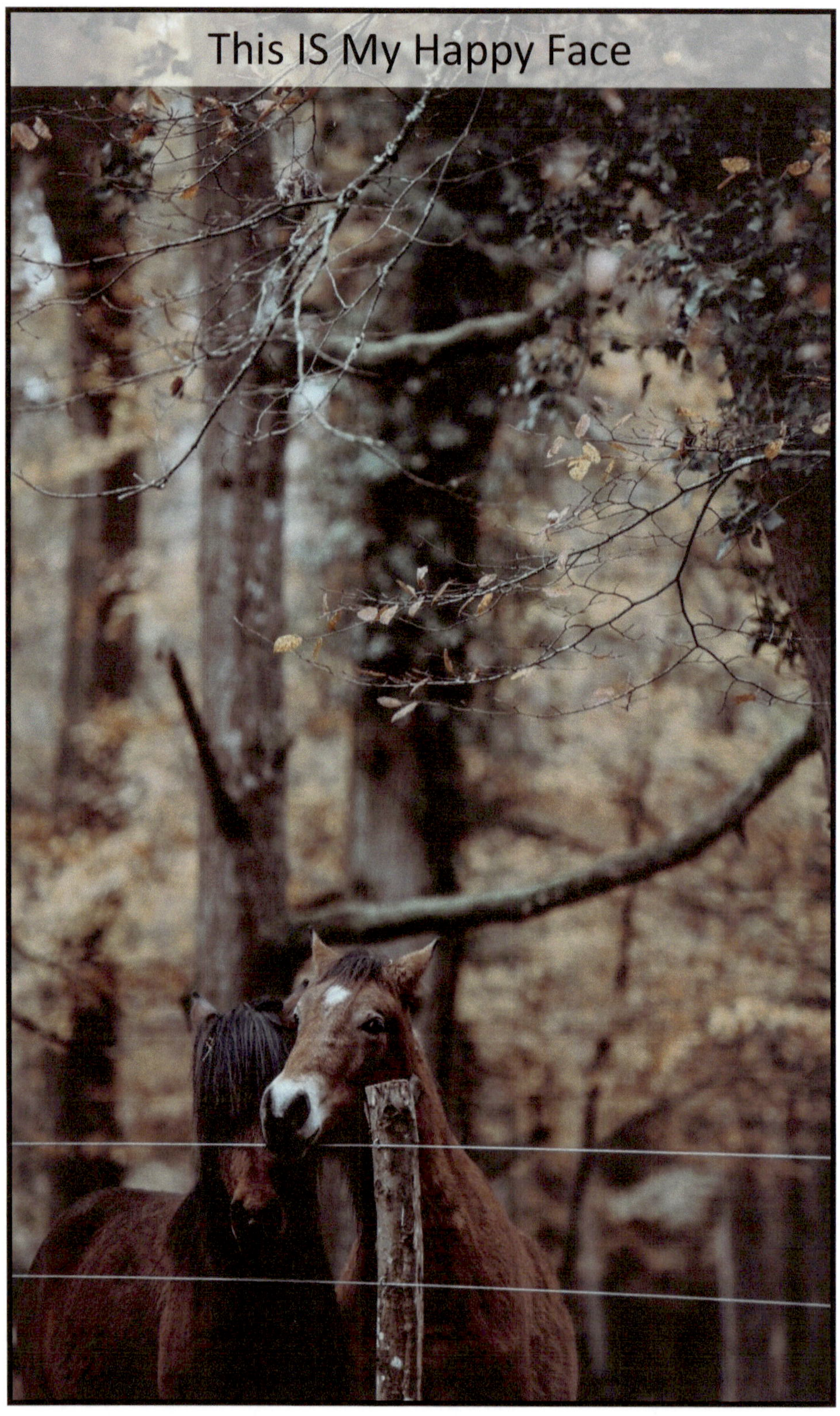

Bliss

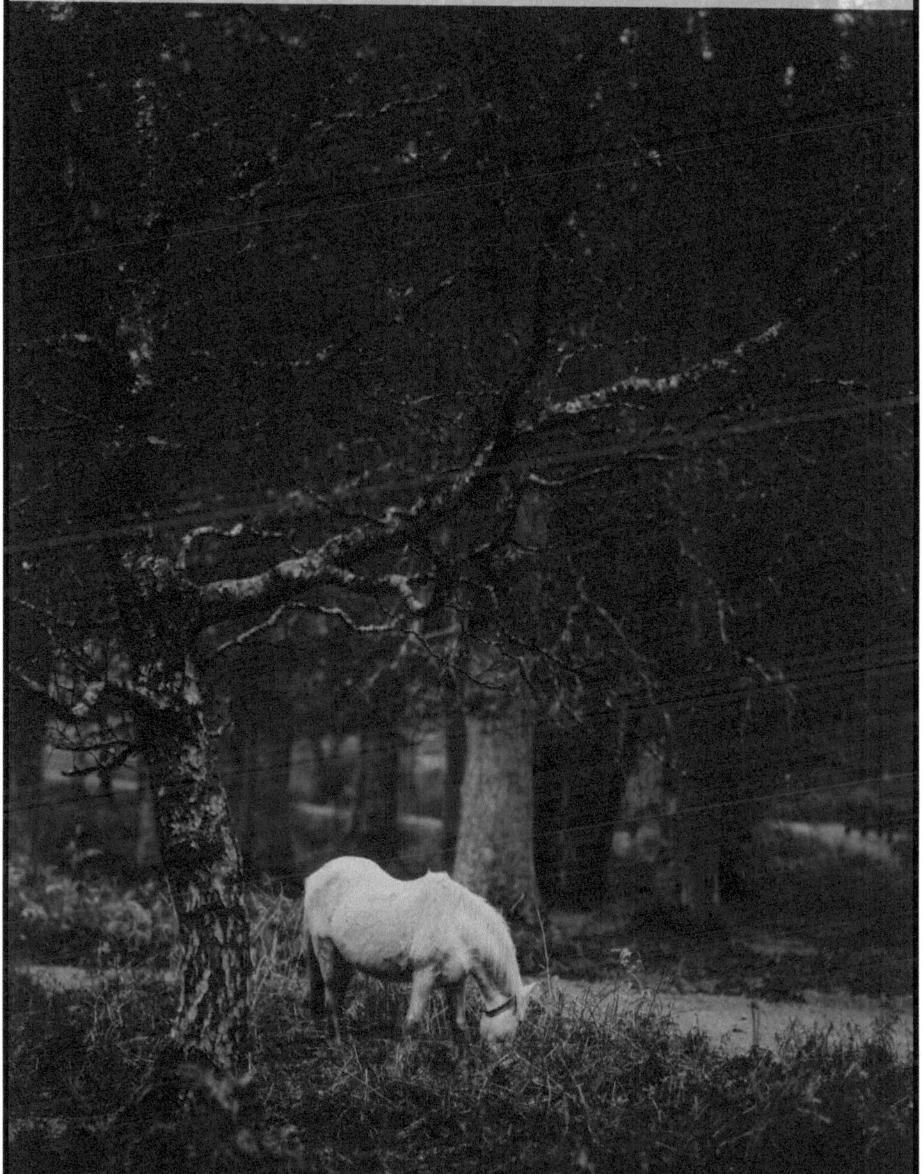

Warm And Sunny

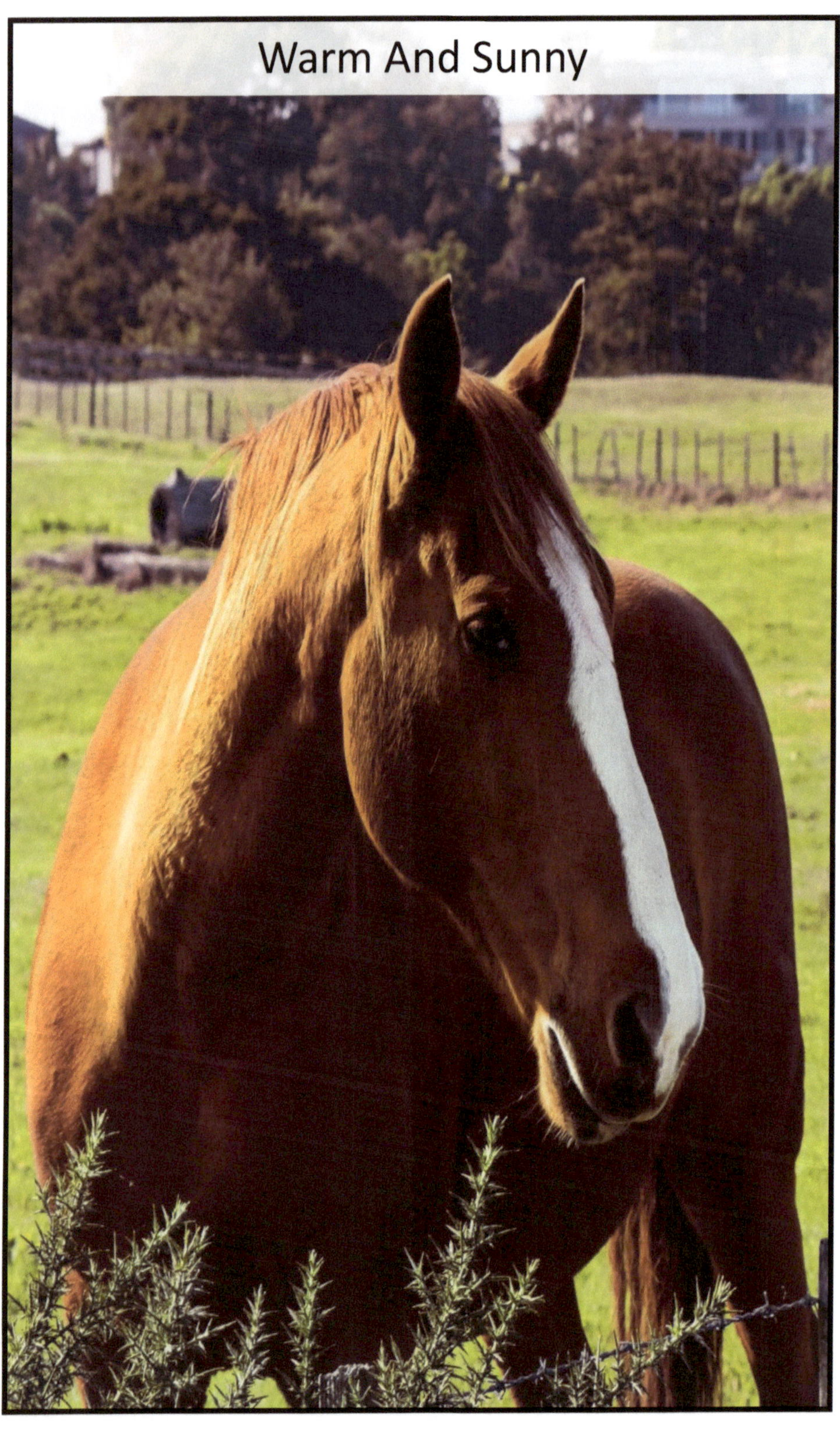

Protection

Having A Bad Hair Day

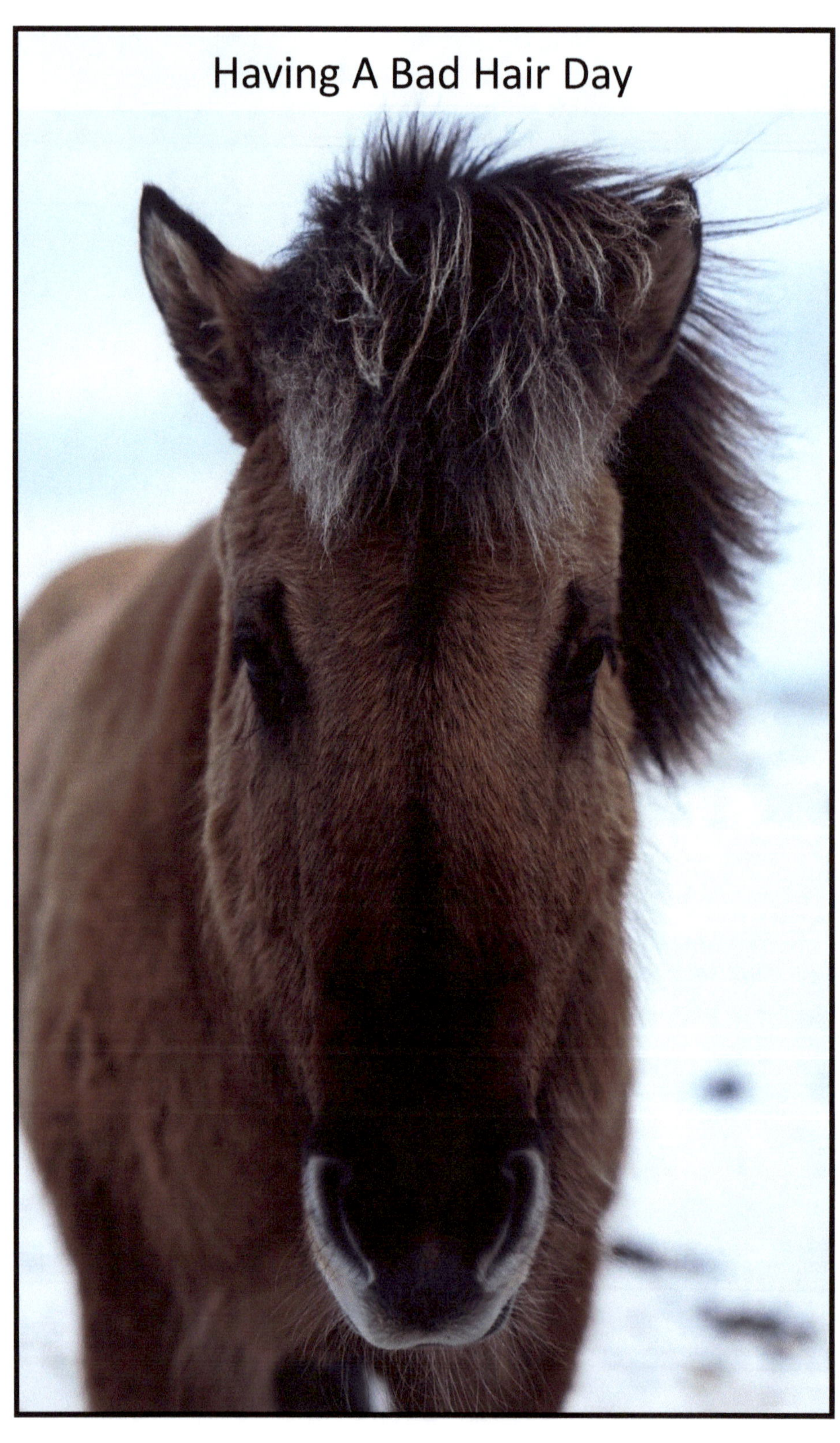

Little But Mighty

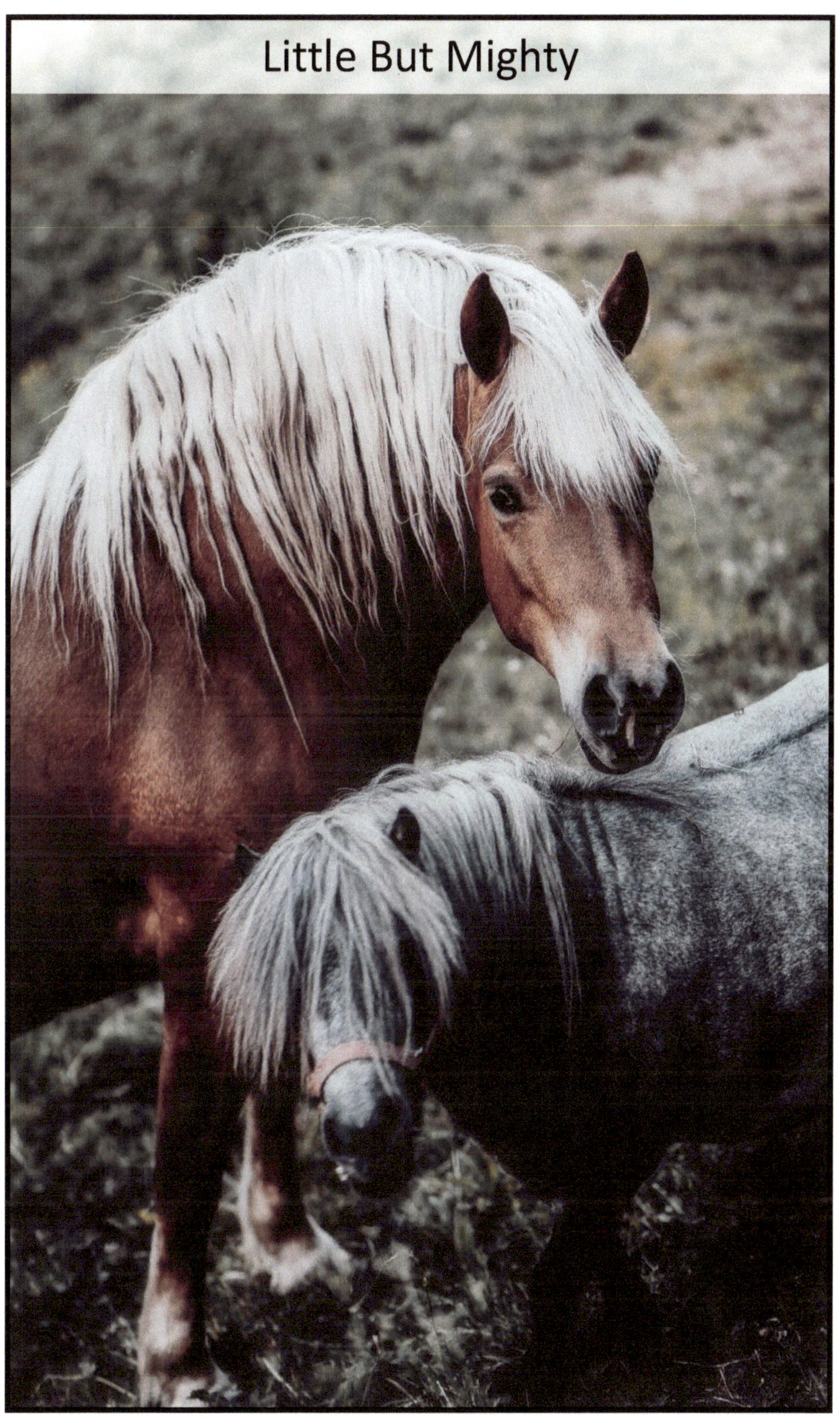

Are You Coming?

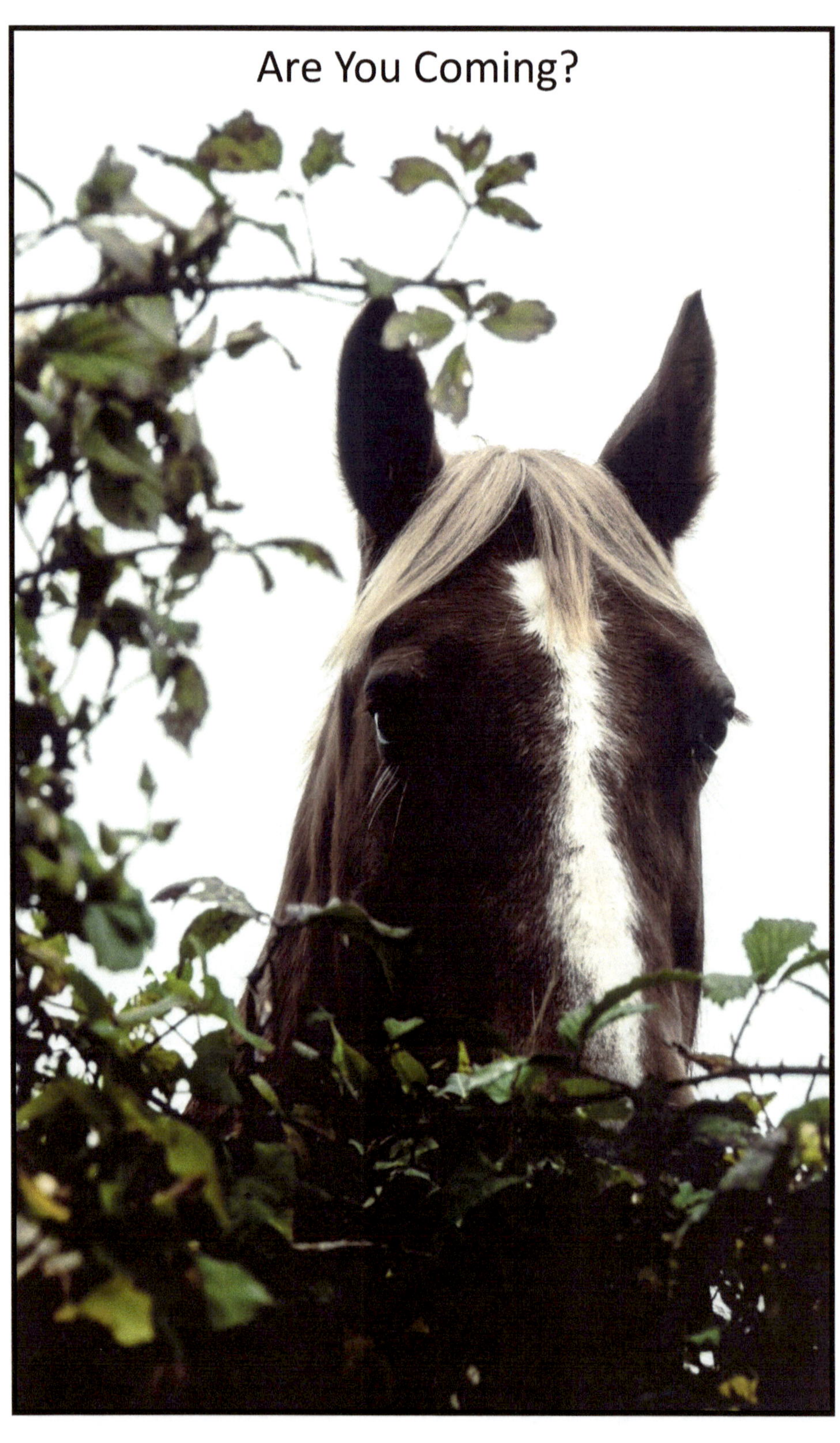

I'm Here For You

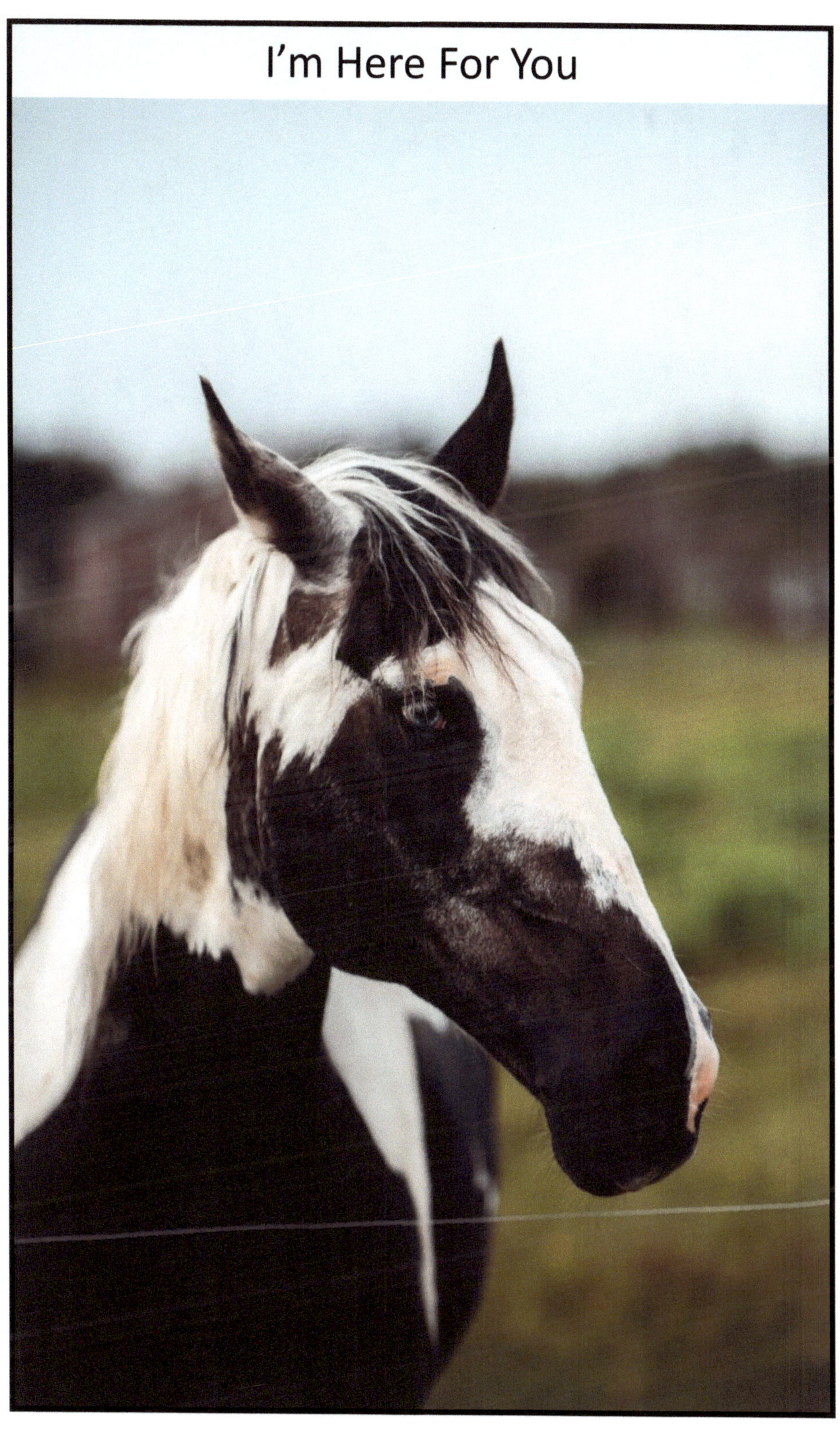

Calm Ocean Breeze

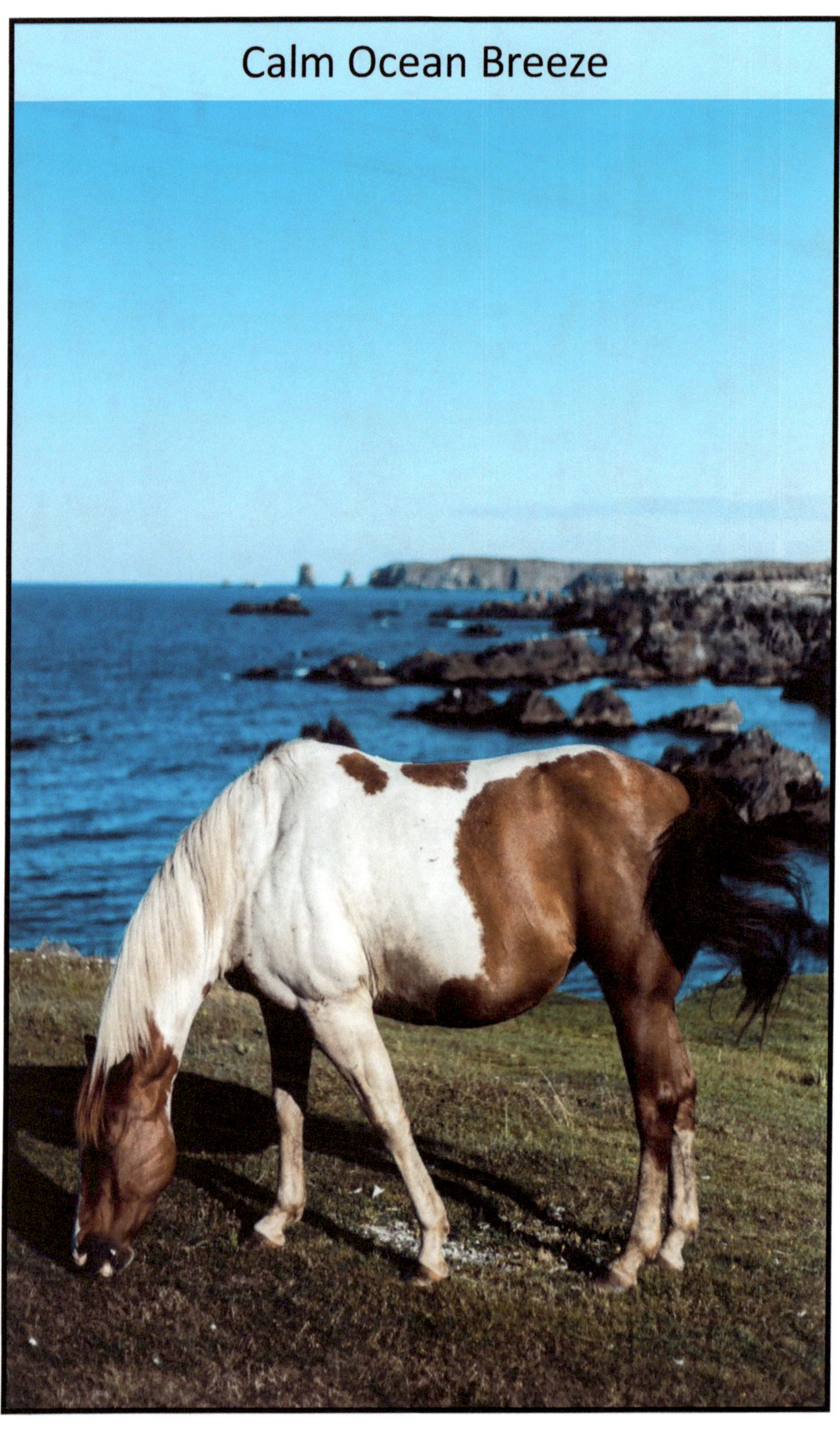

Green Pastures

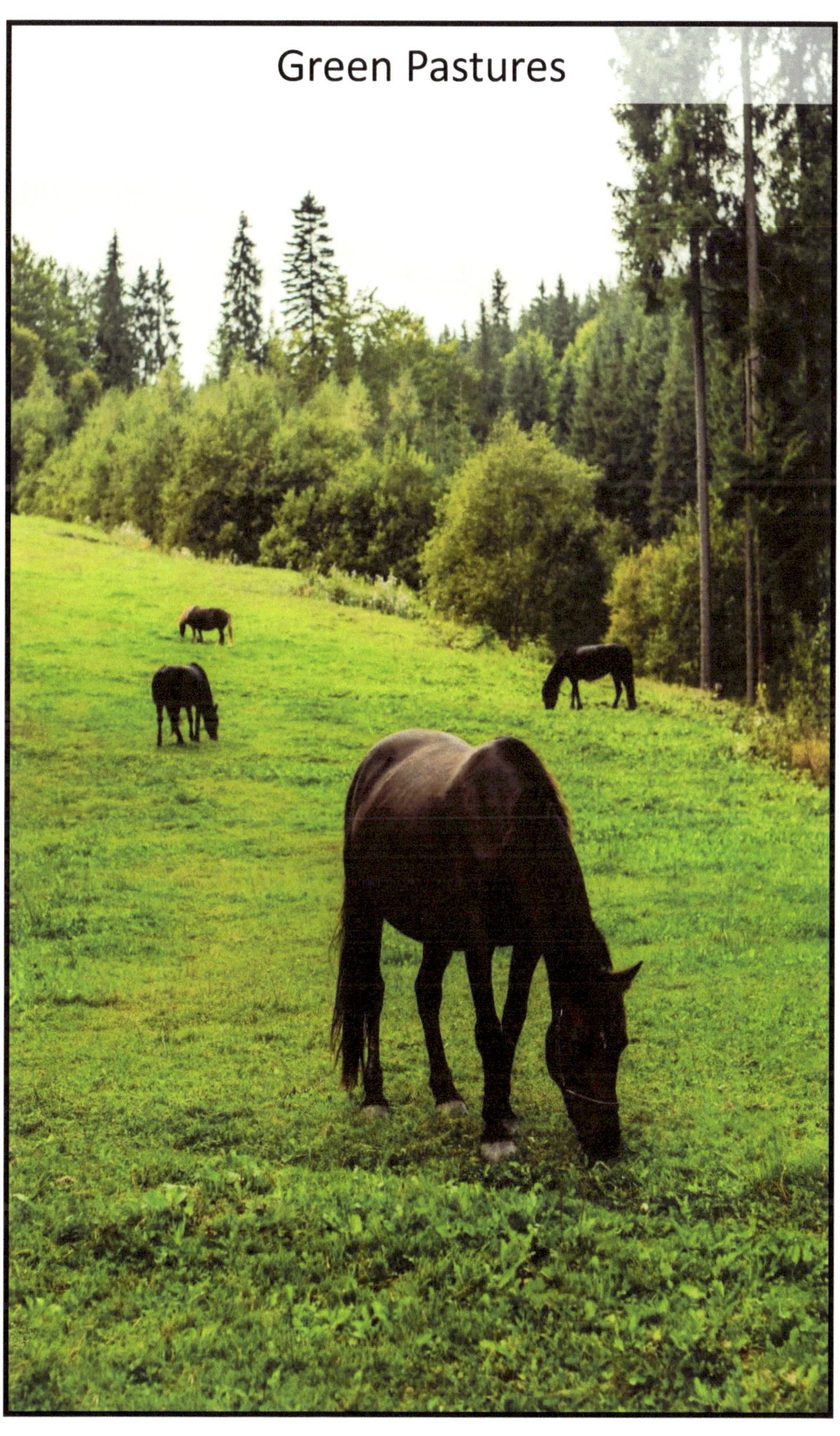

Time For A Ride?

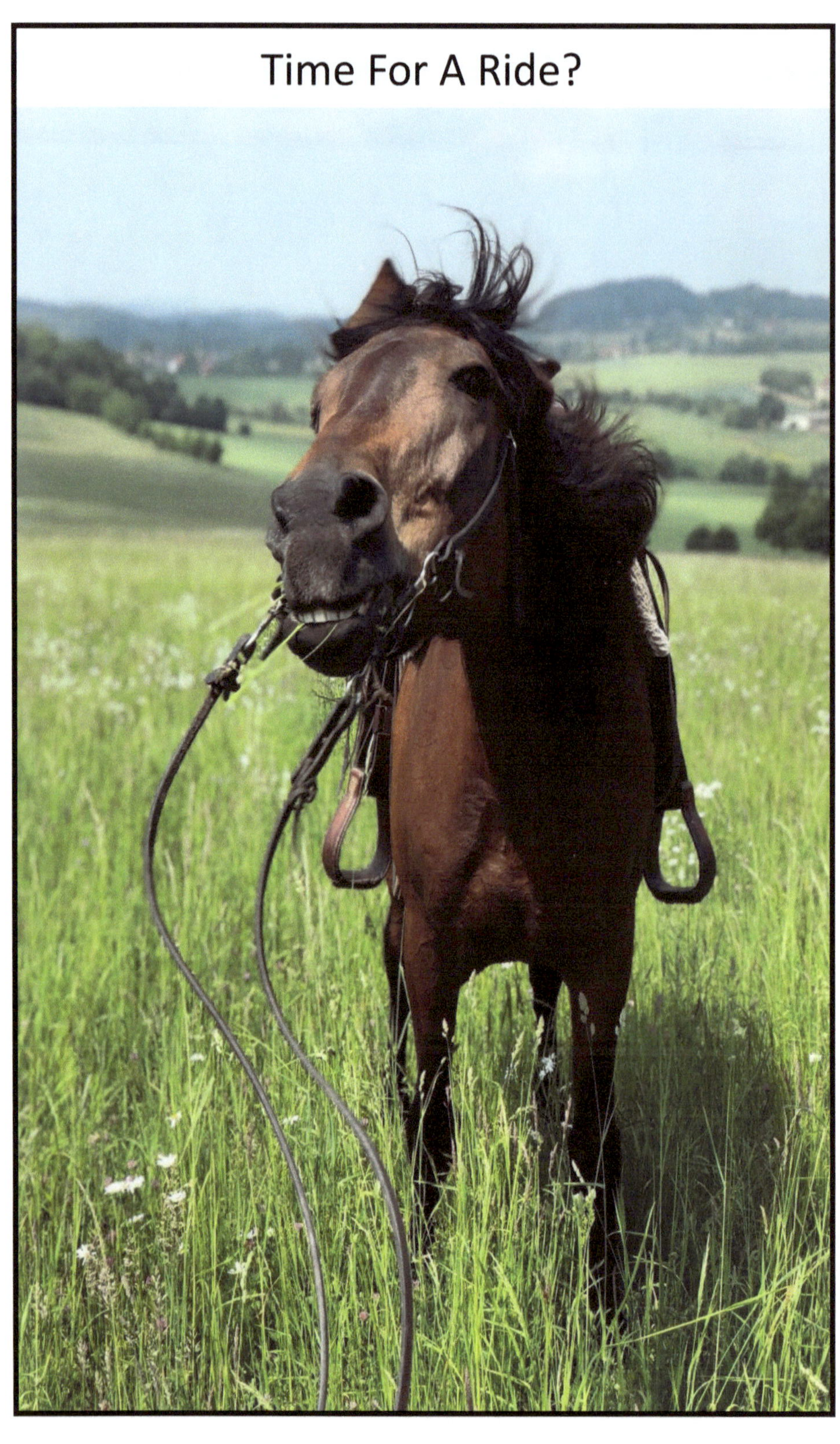

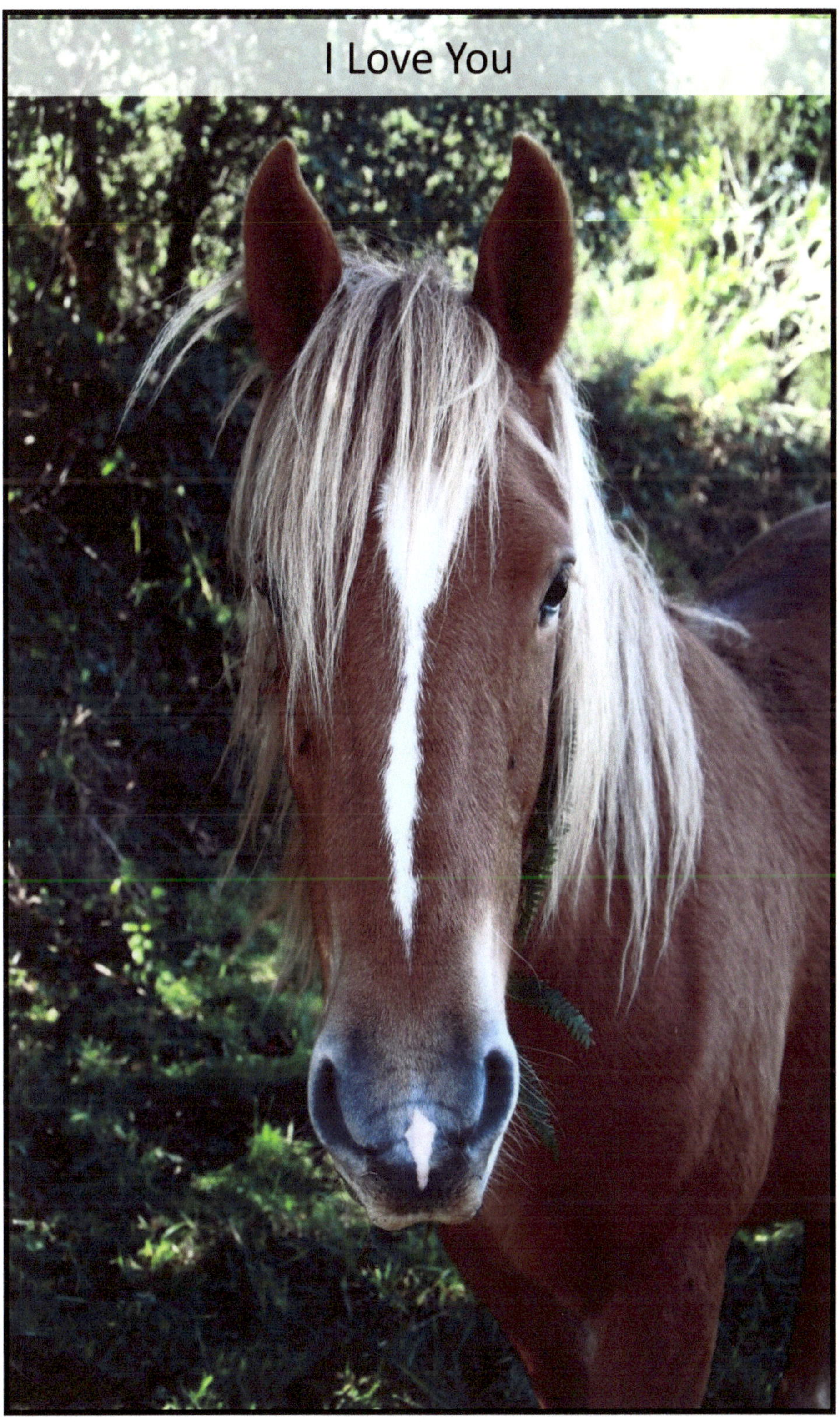

I Love You

Dawn

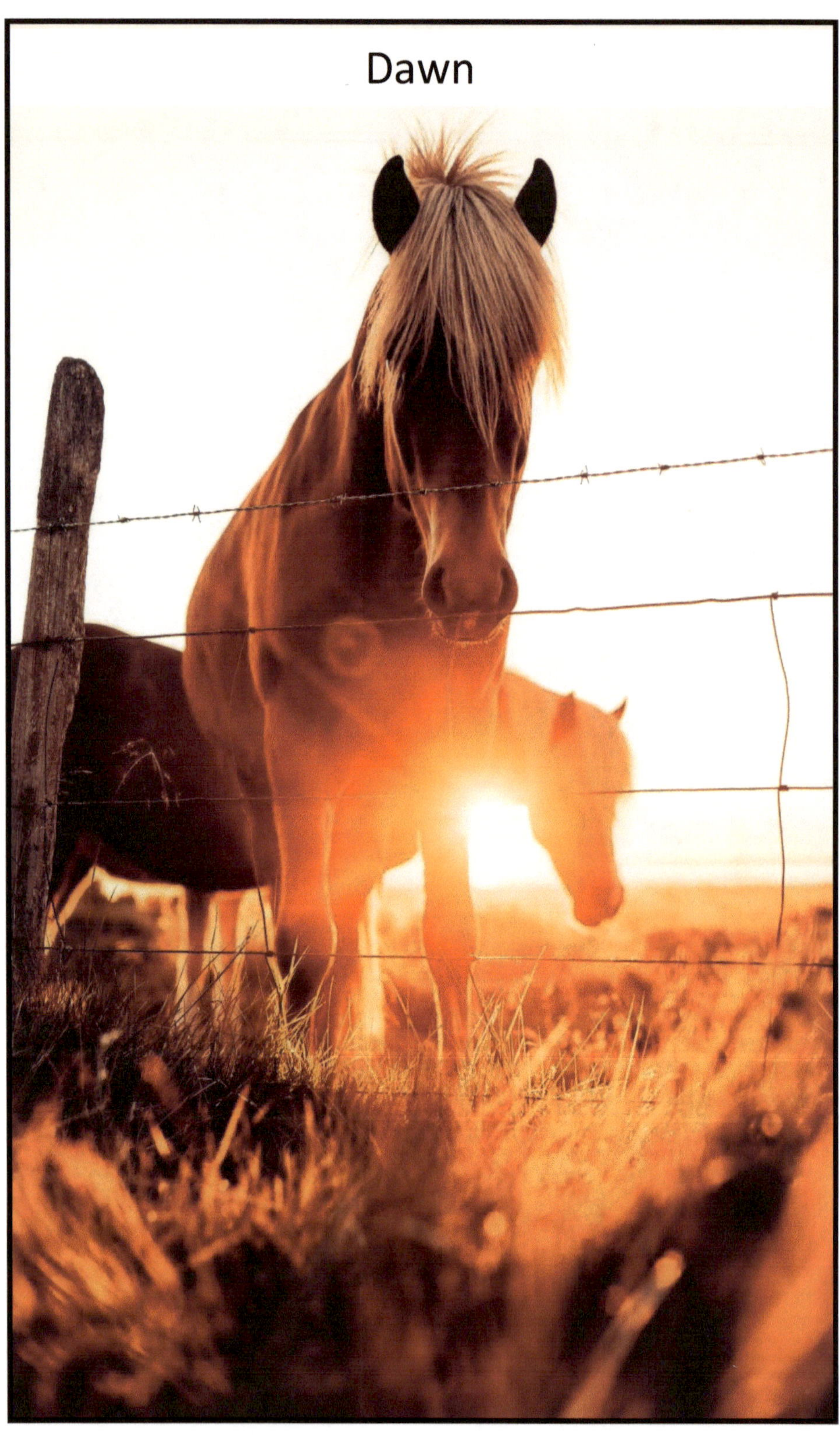

This Is My Spot

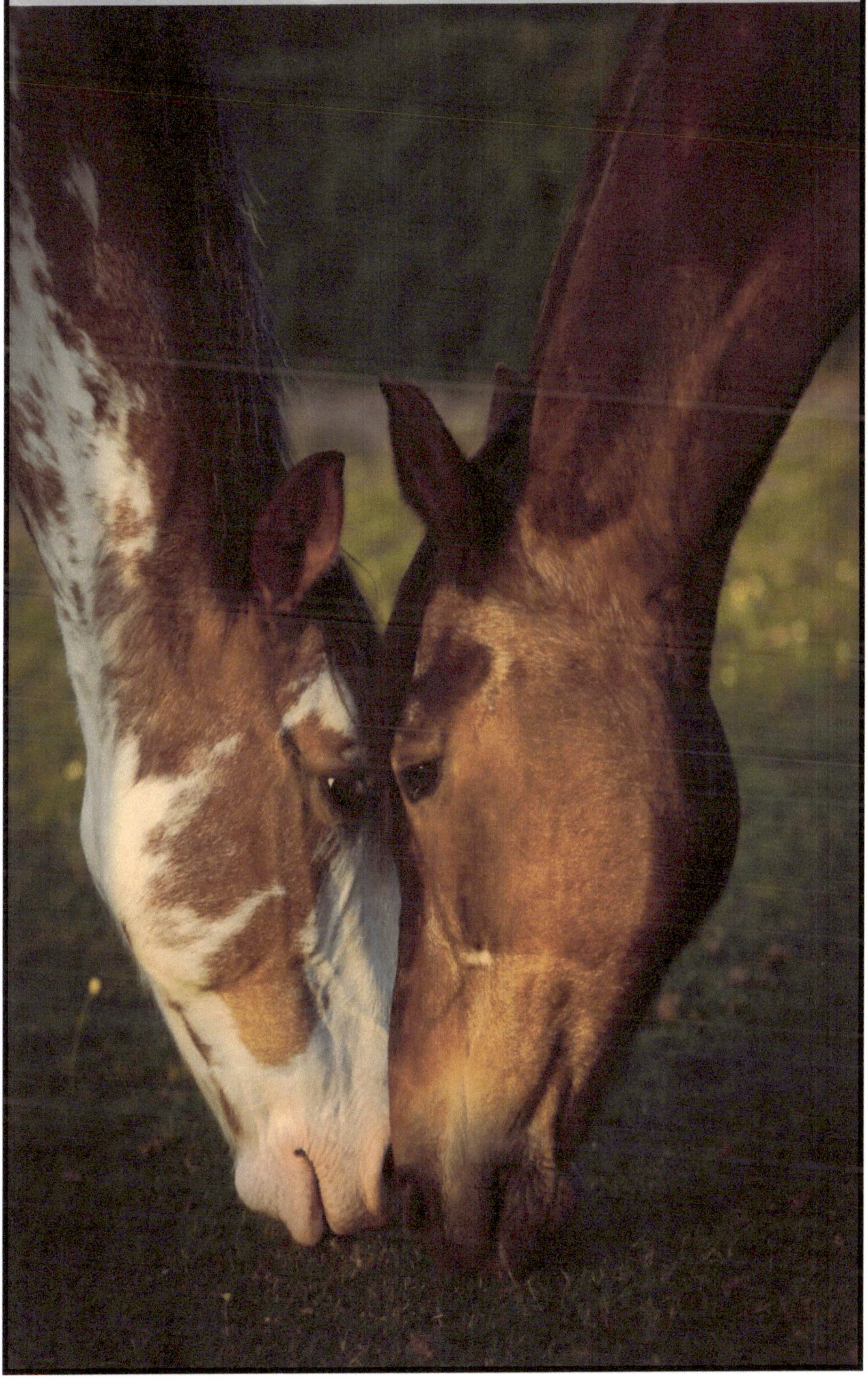

Why Are You Yelling At Me?

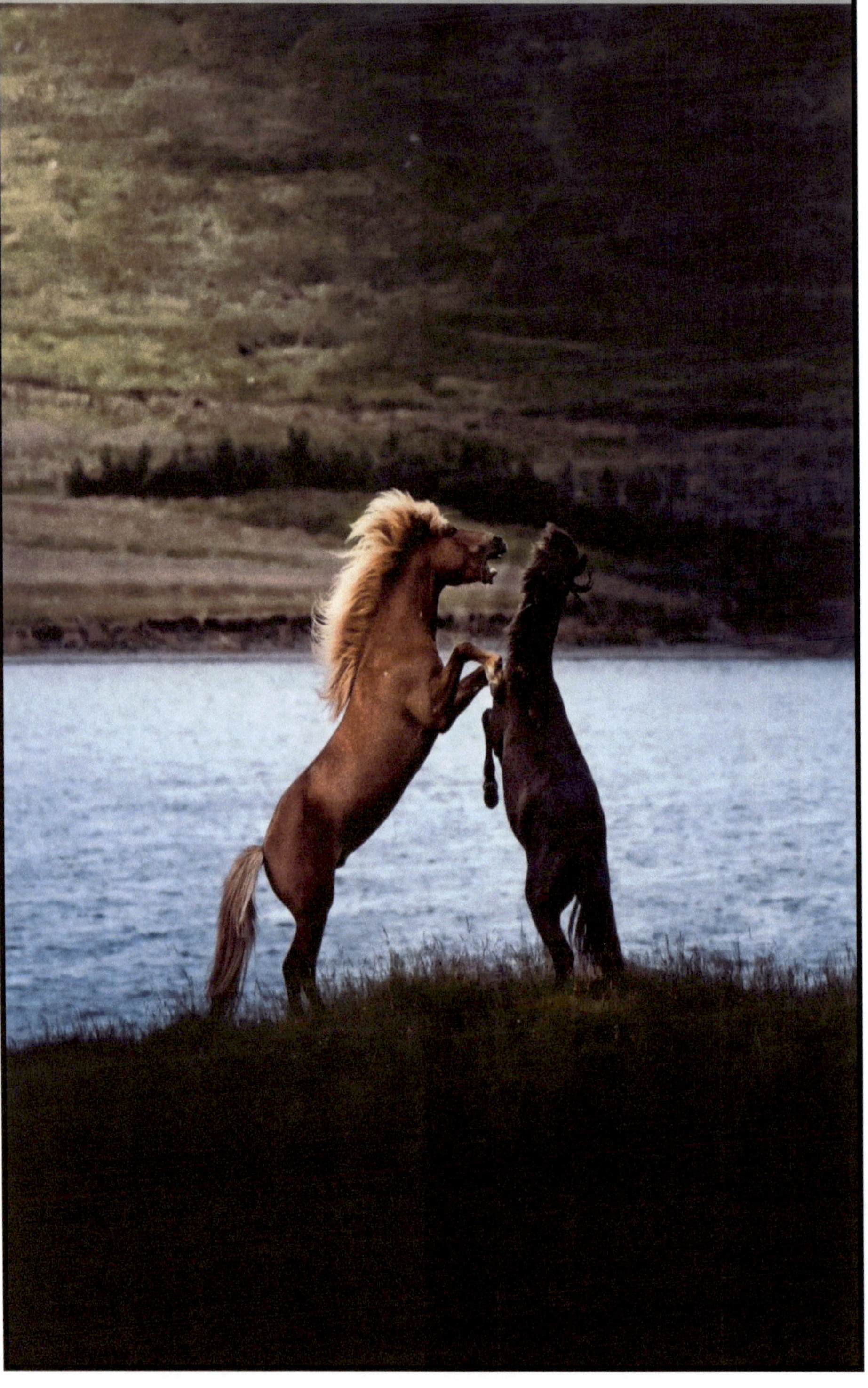

Icy Cold Morning

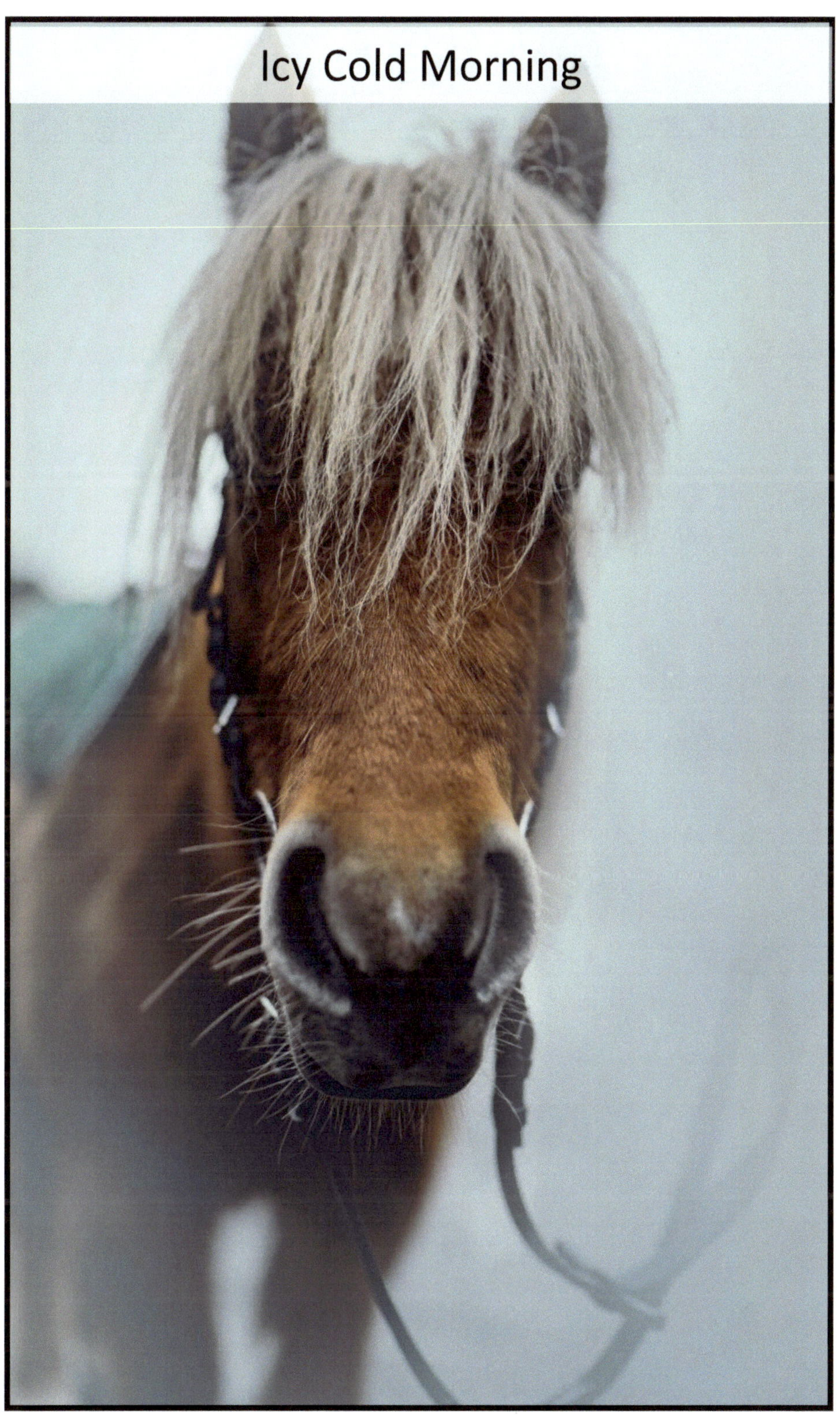

Hello Bright Eyes

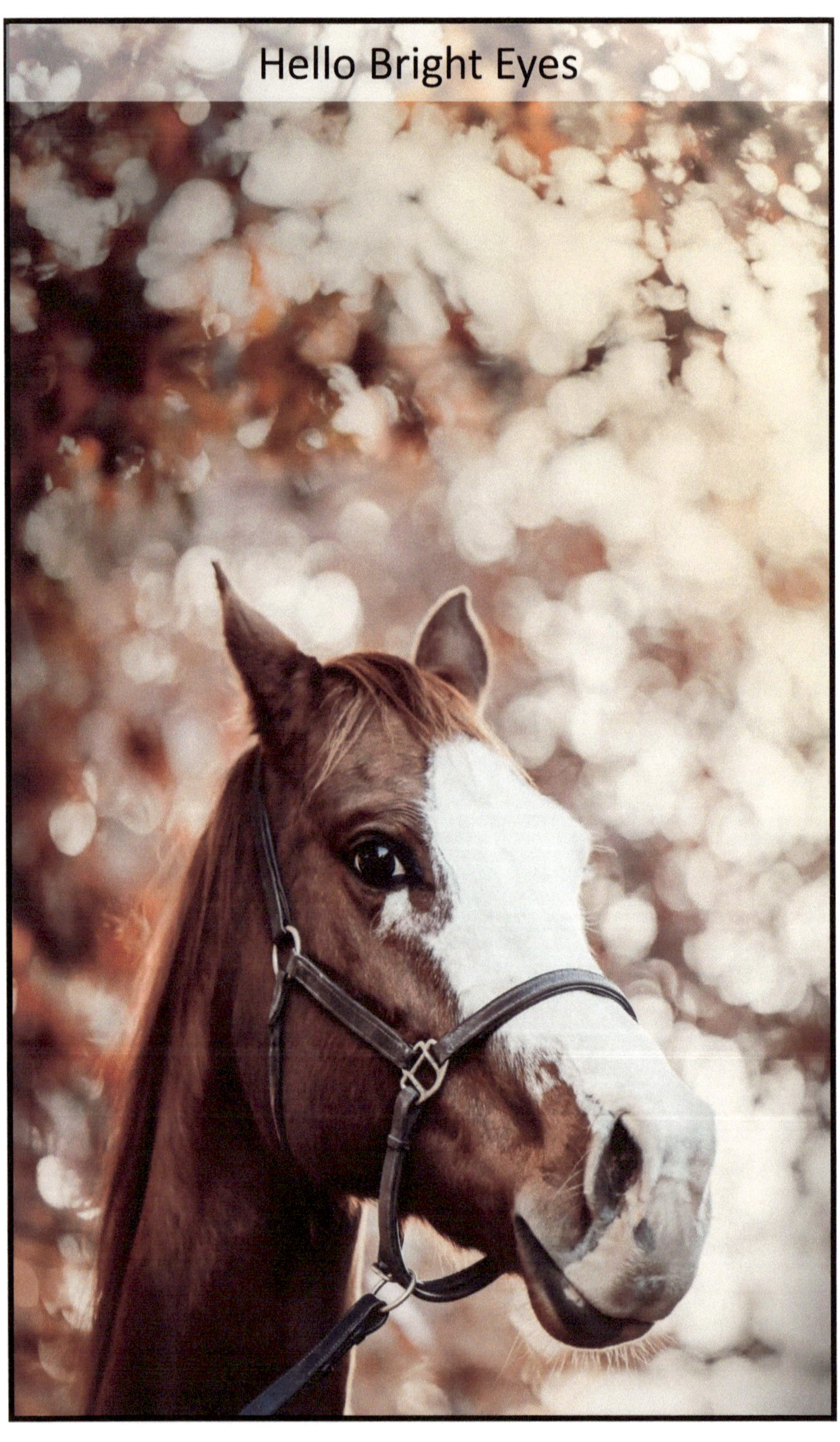

Is It Dinner Yet?

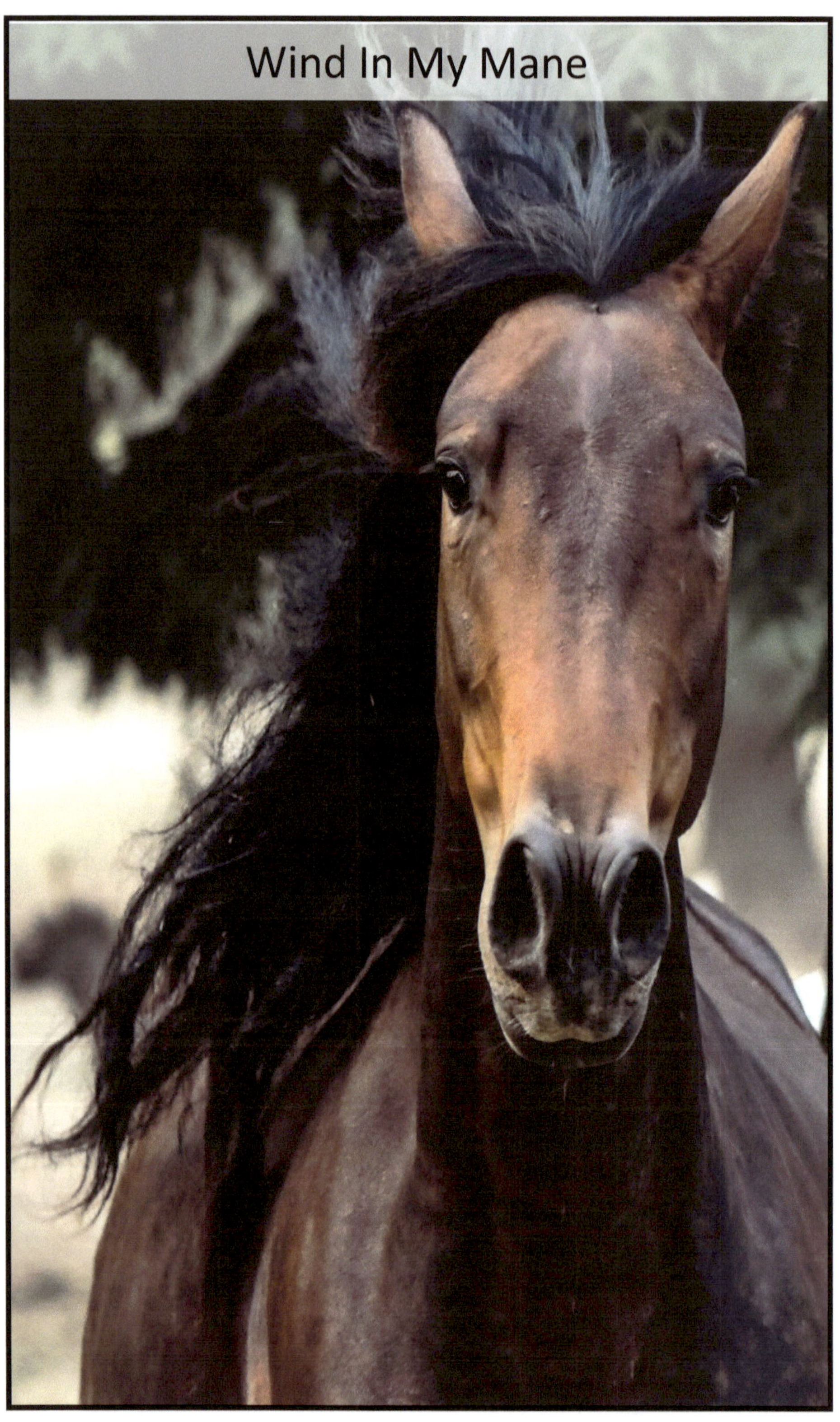

Wind In My Mane

Thinking Of You

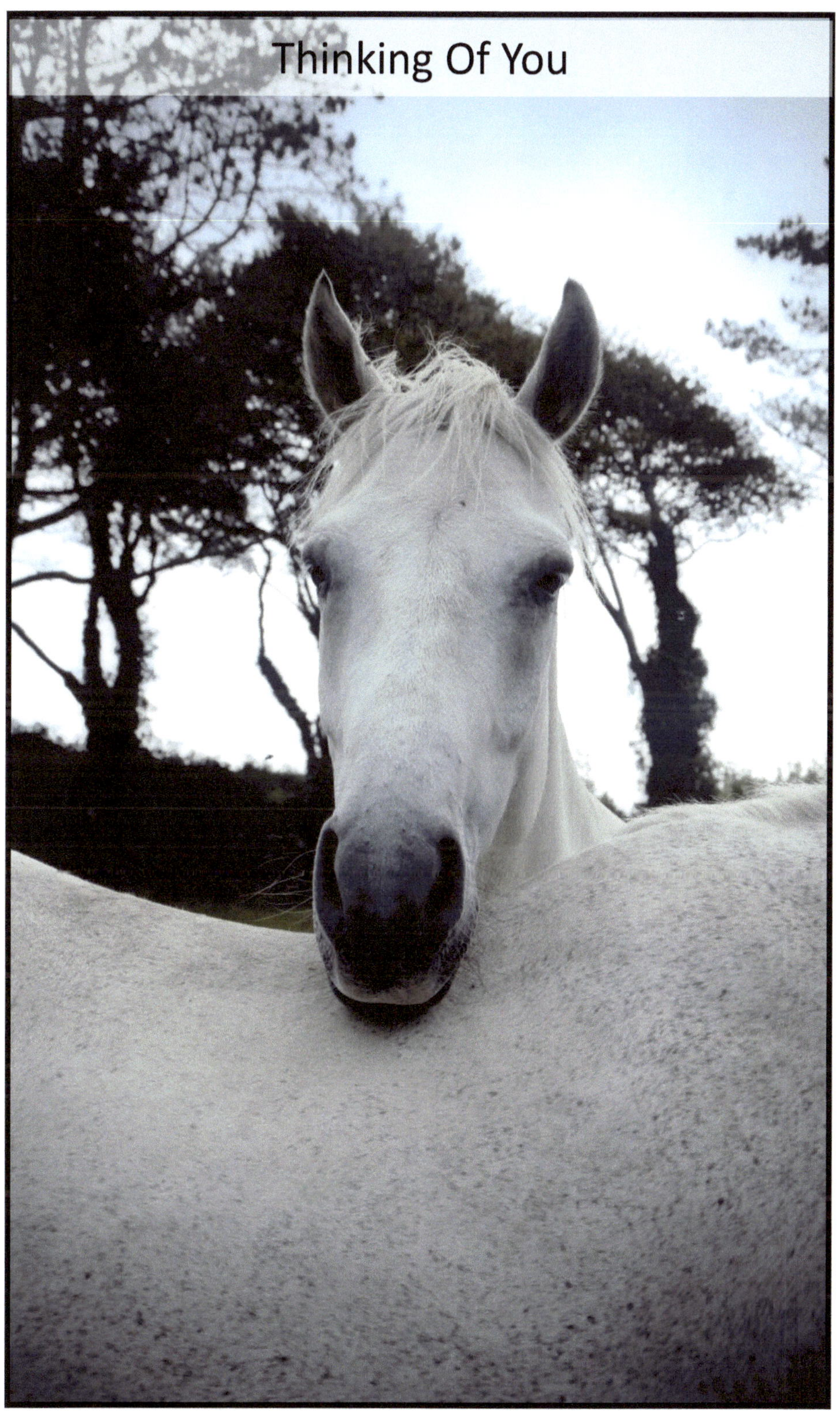

Up Hill, Both Ways, In The Snow

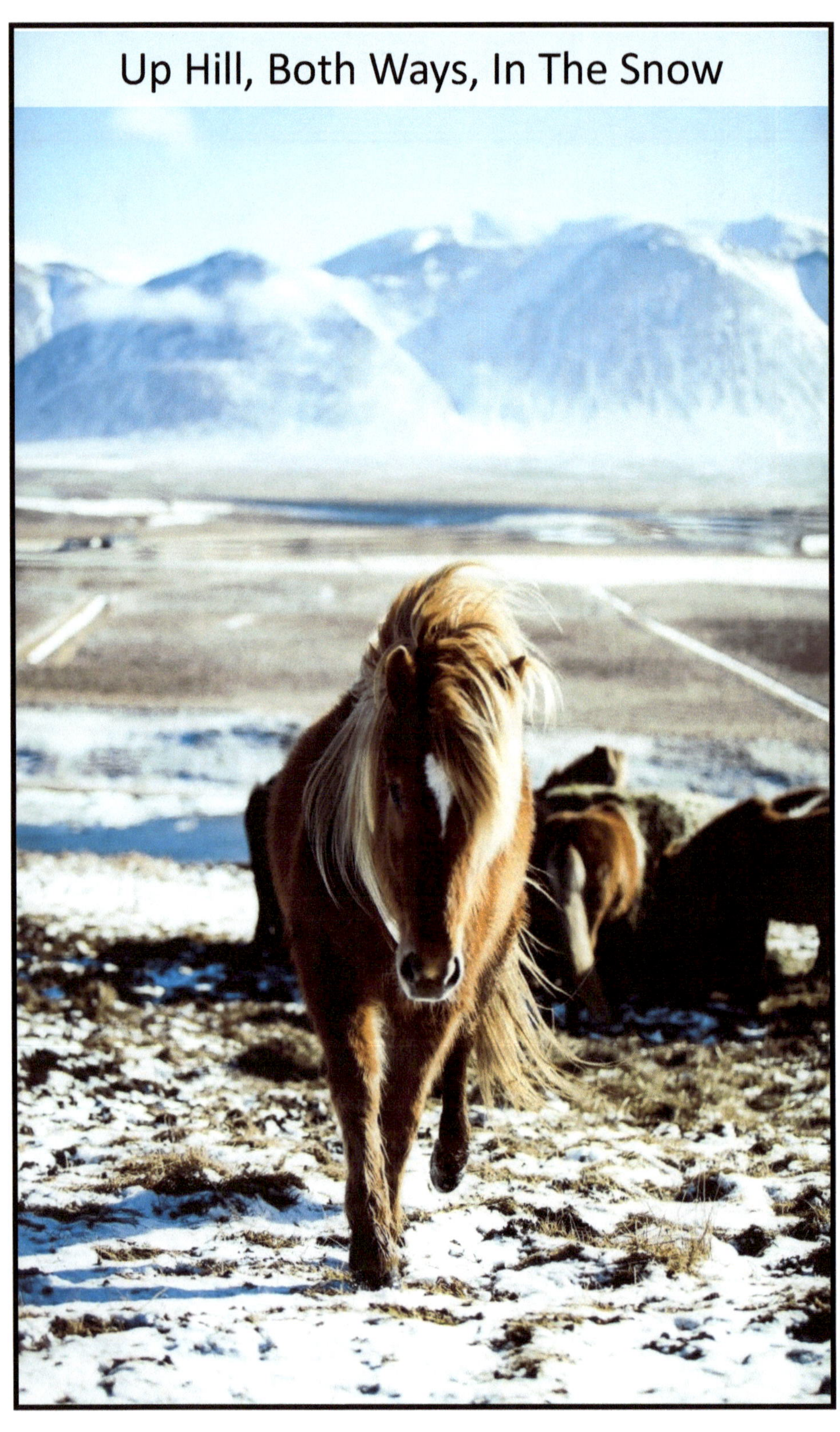

Yes, I'm A Happy Boy

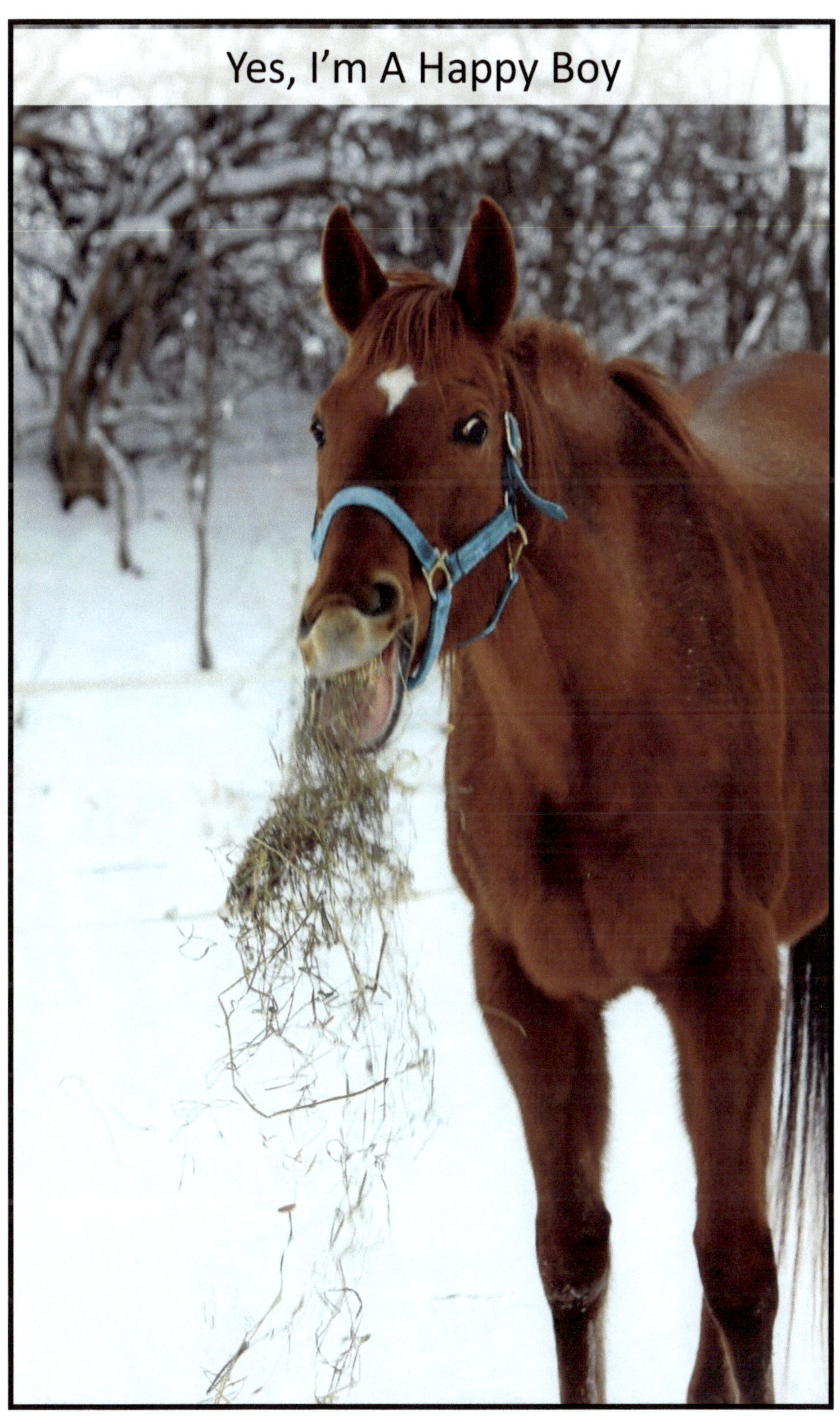

Patriotic

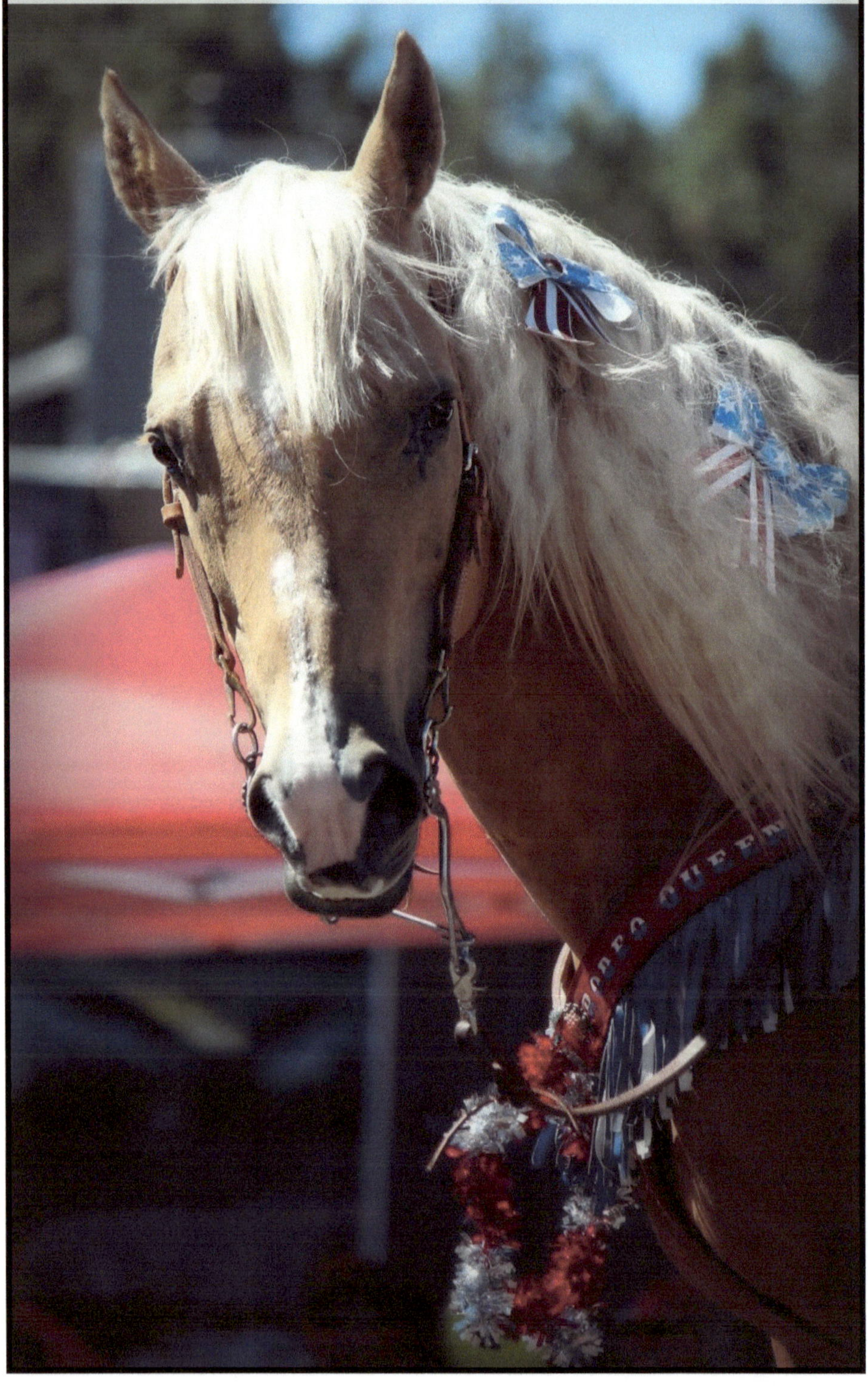

Seeing Double

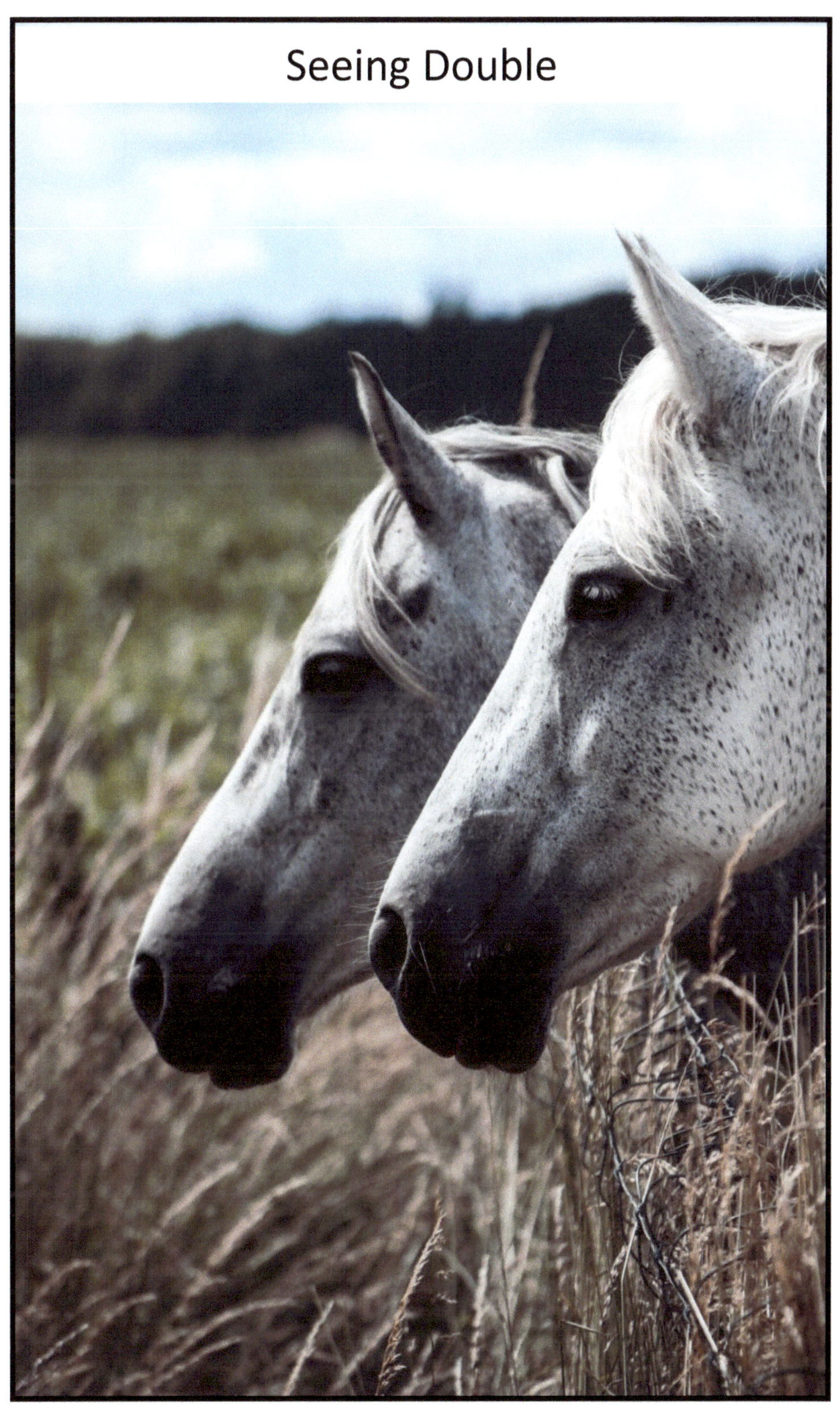

Snow Day

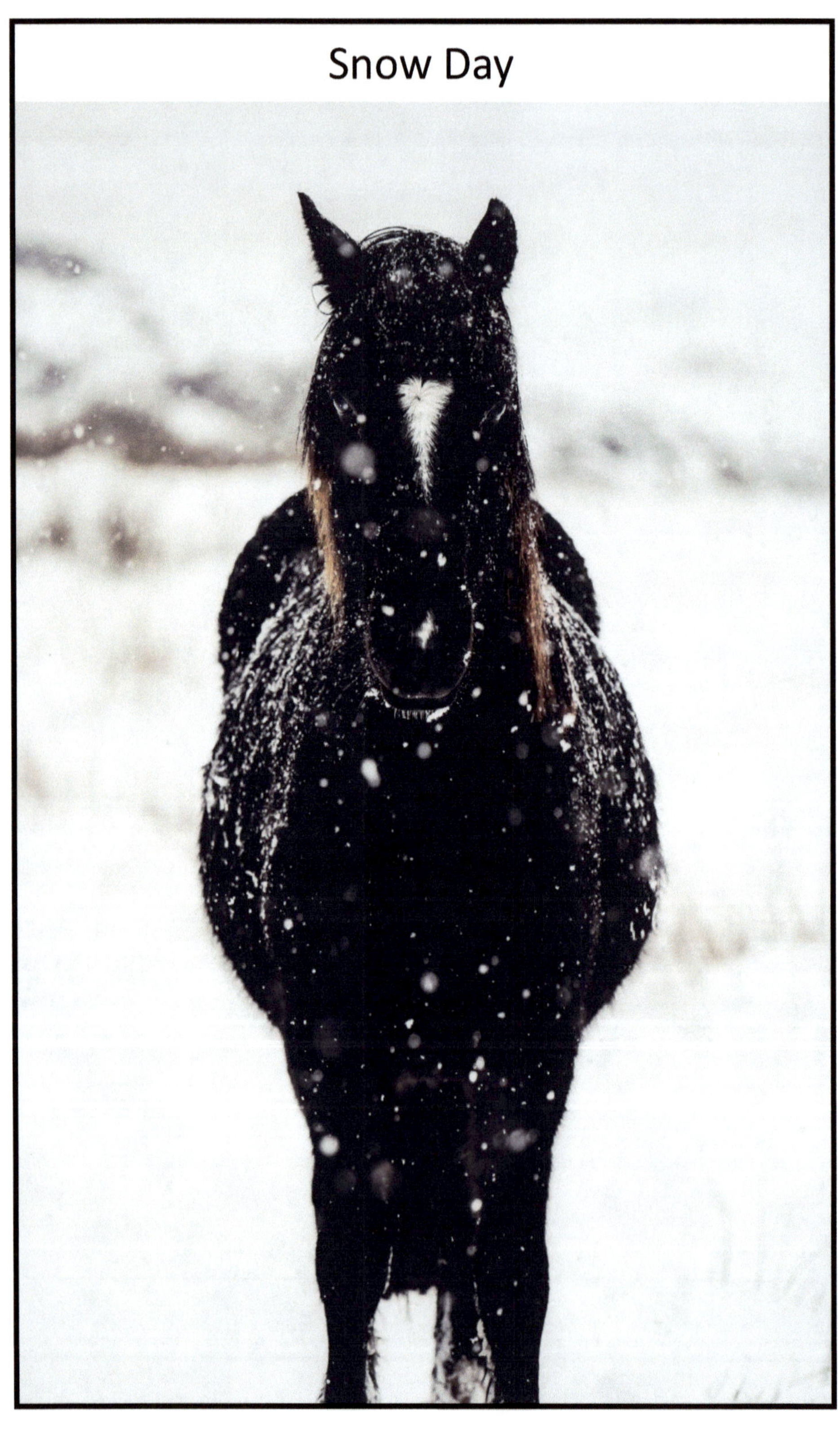

My Happy Place

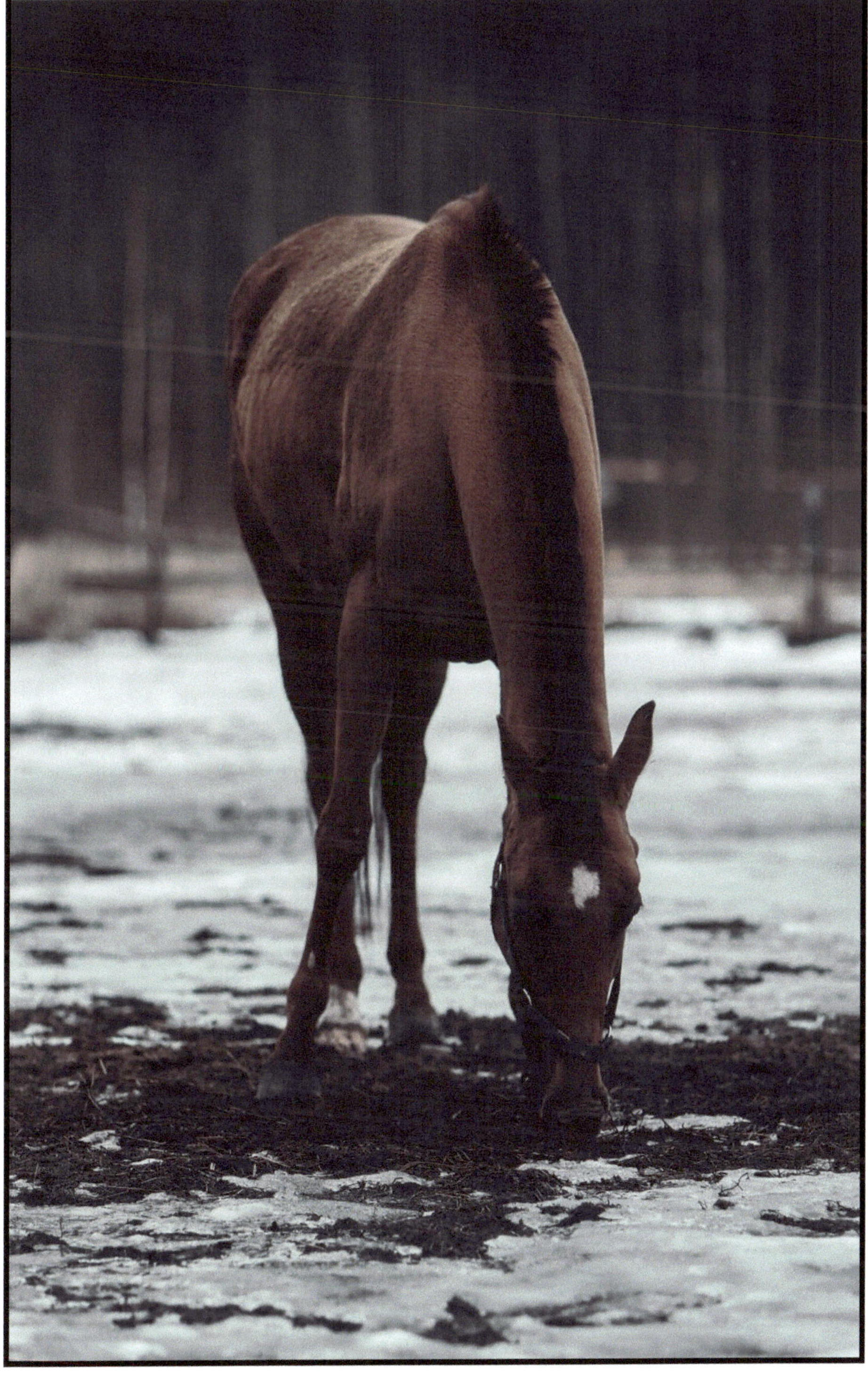

Breakfast

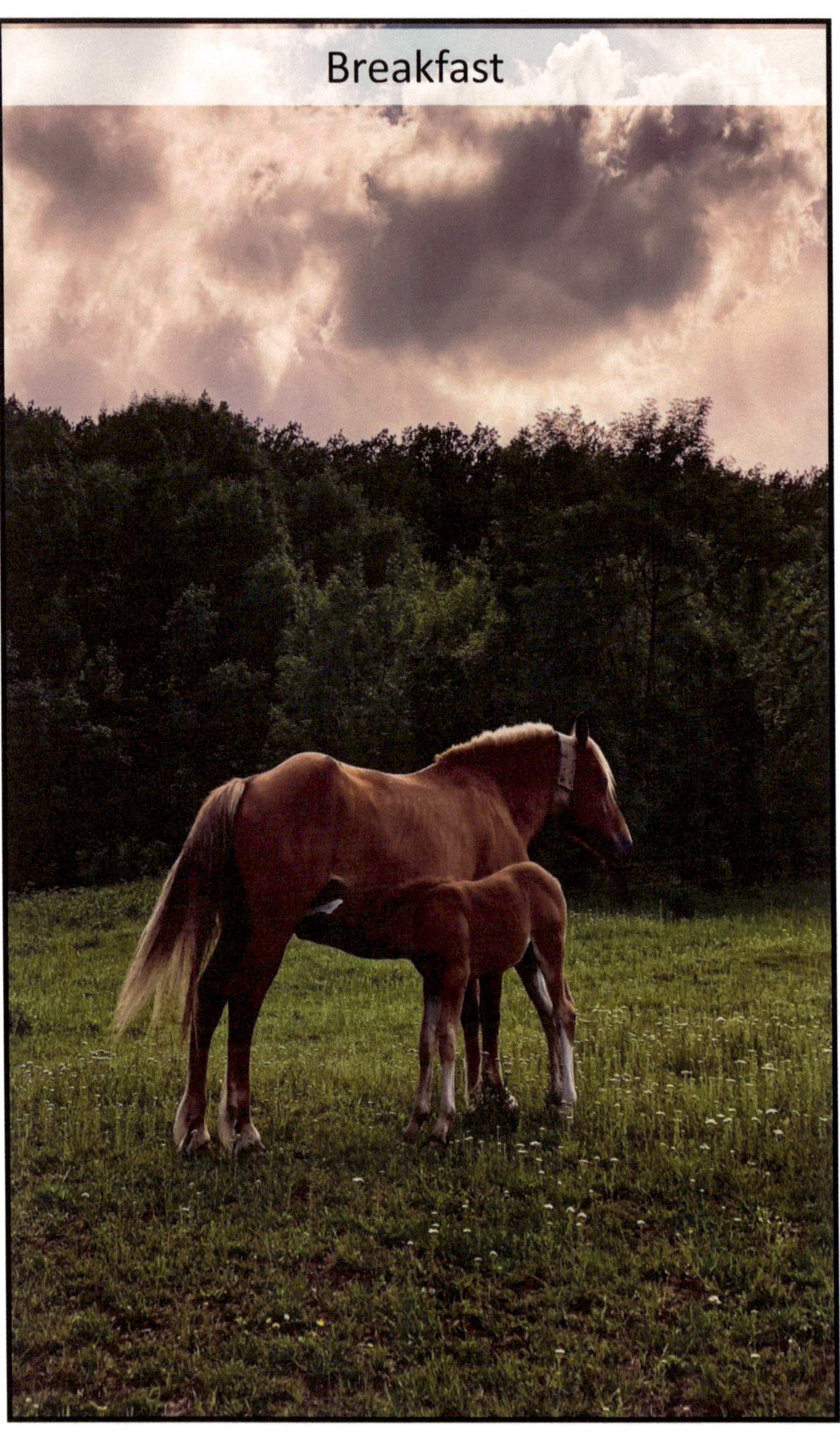

Breakfast

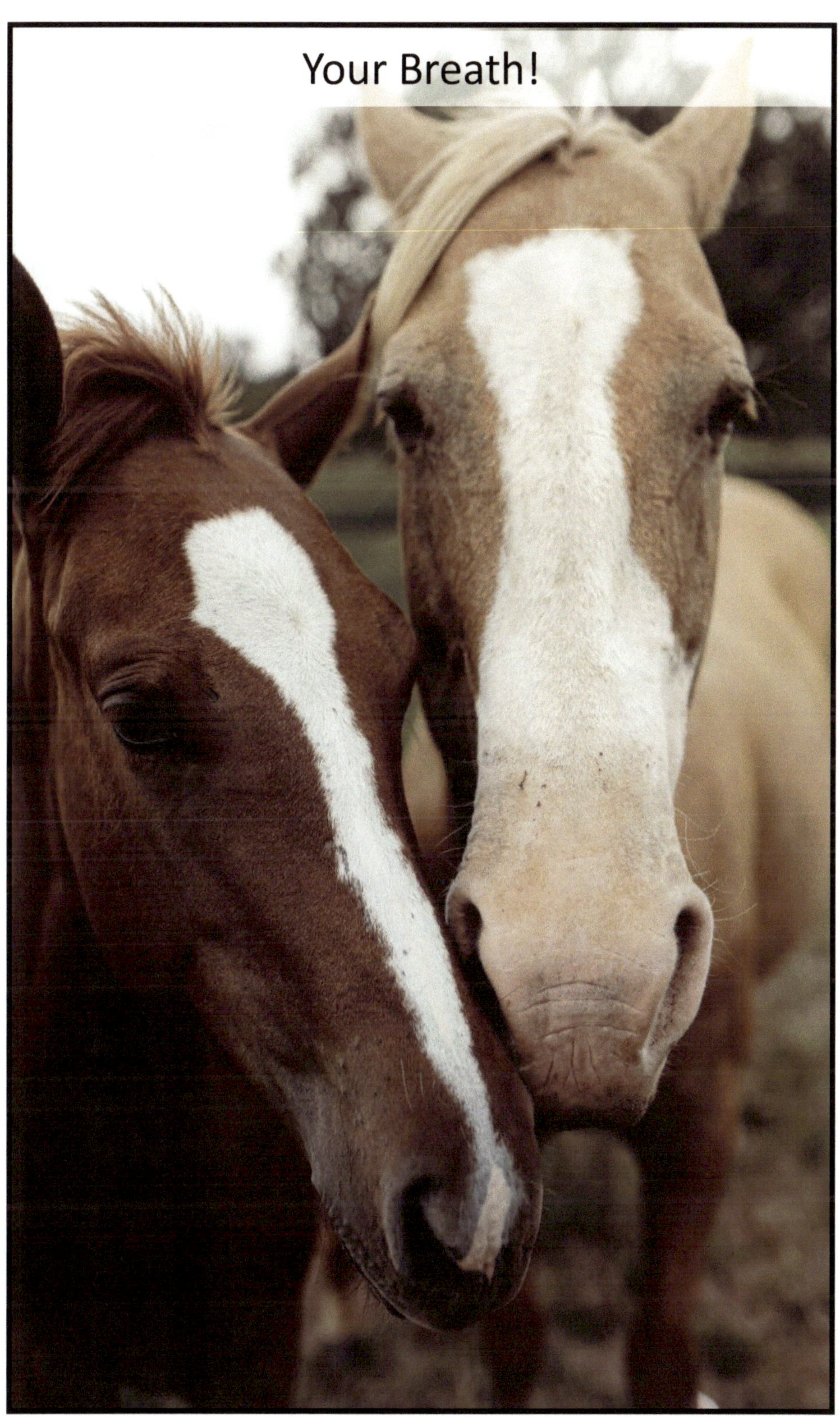

Your Breath!

This Is My Good Side

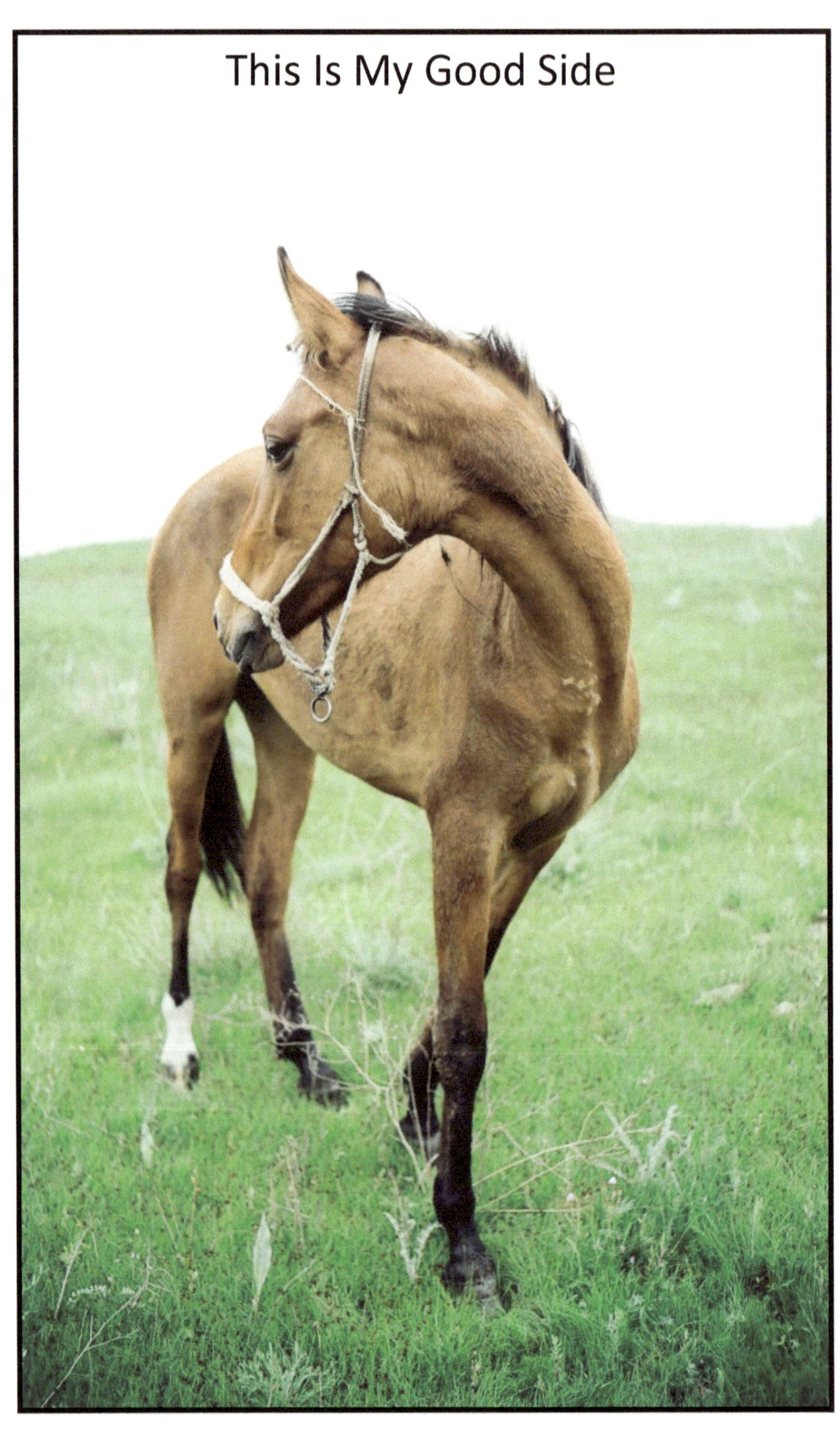

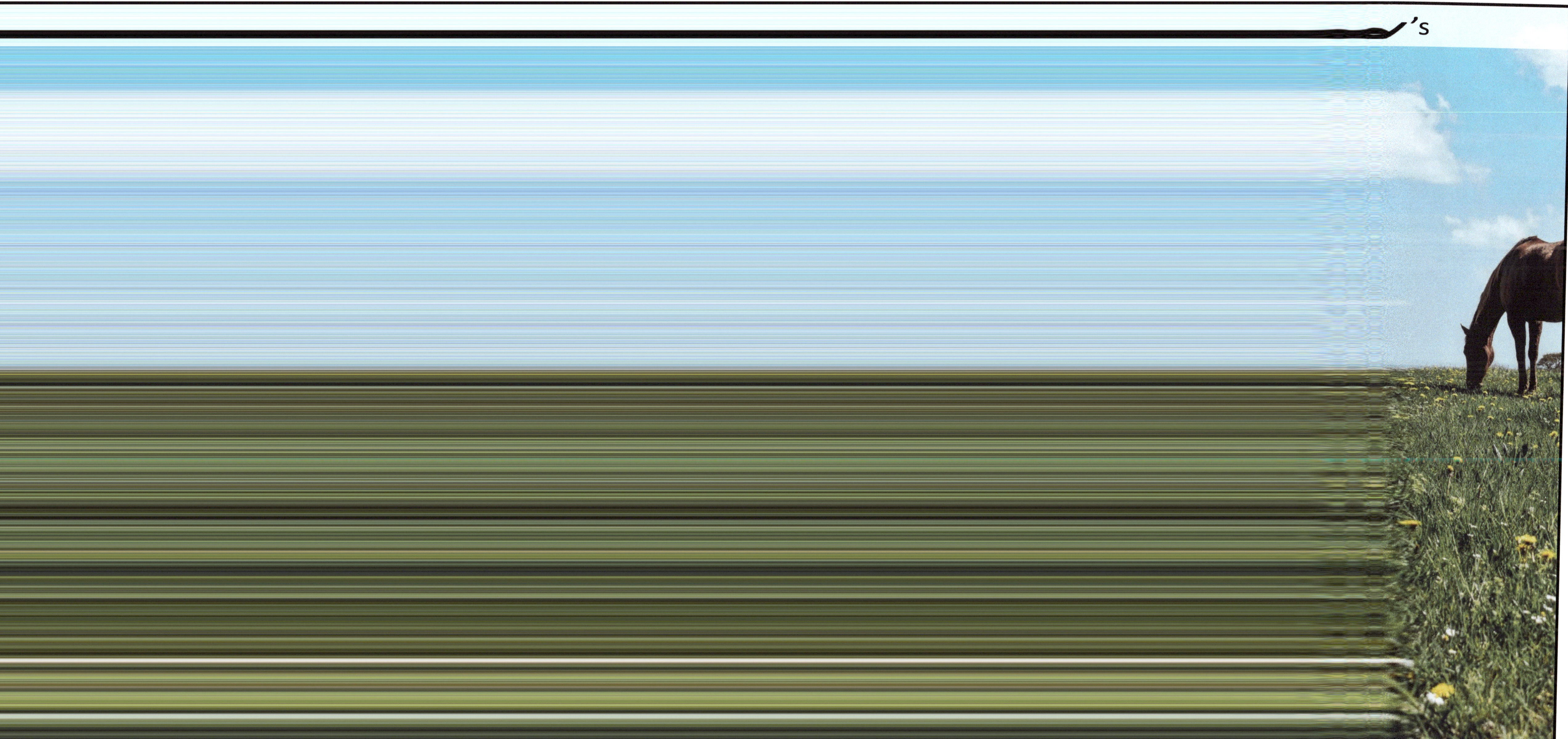

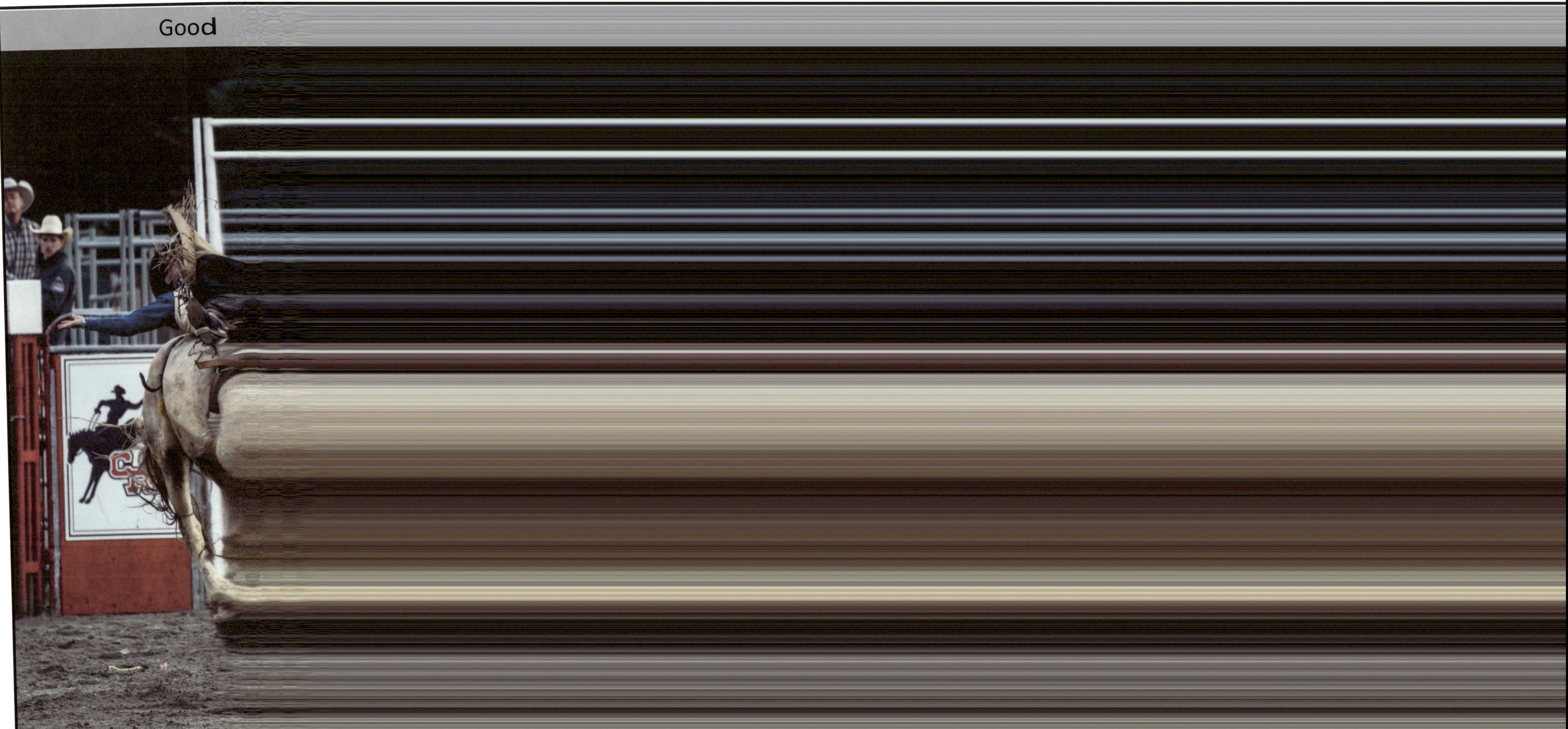
Good

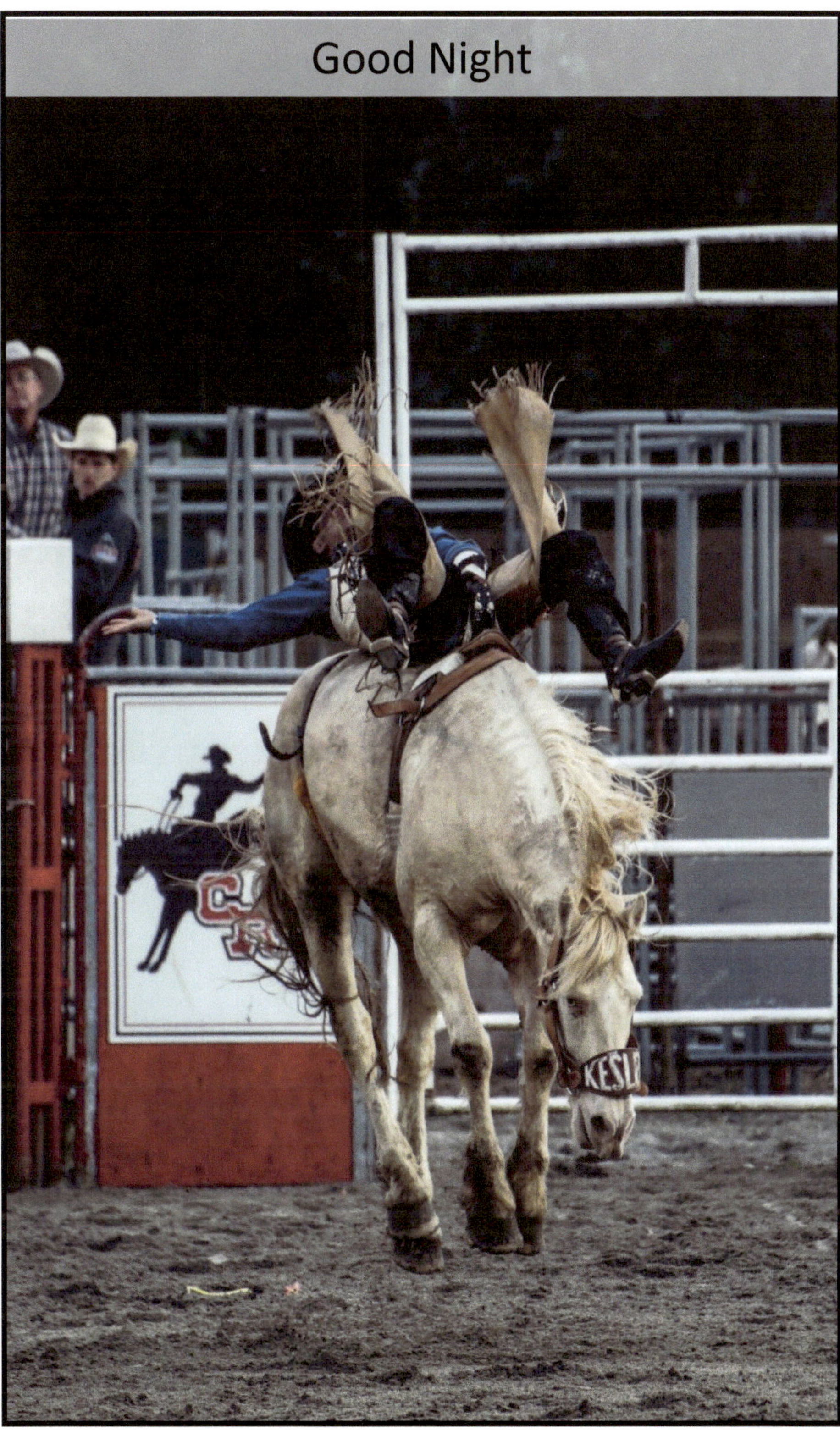

KESLE

Spring Allergy's

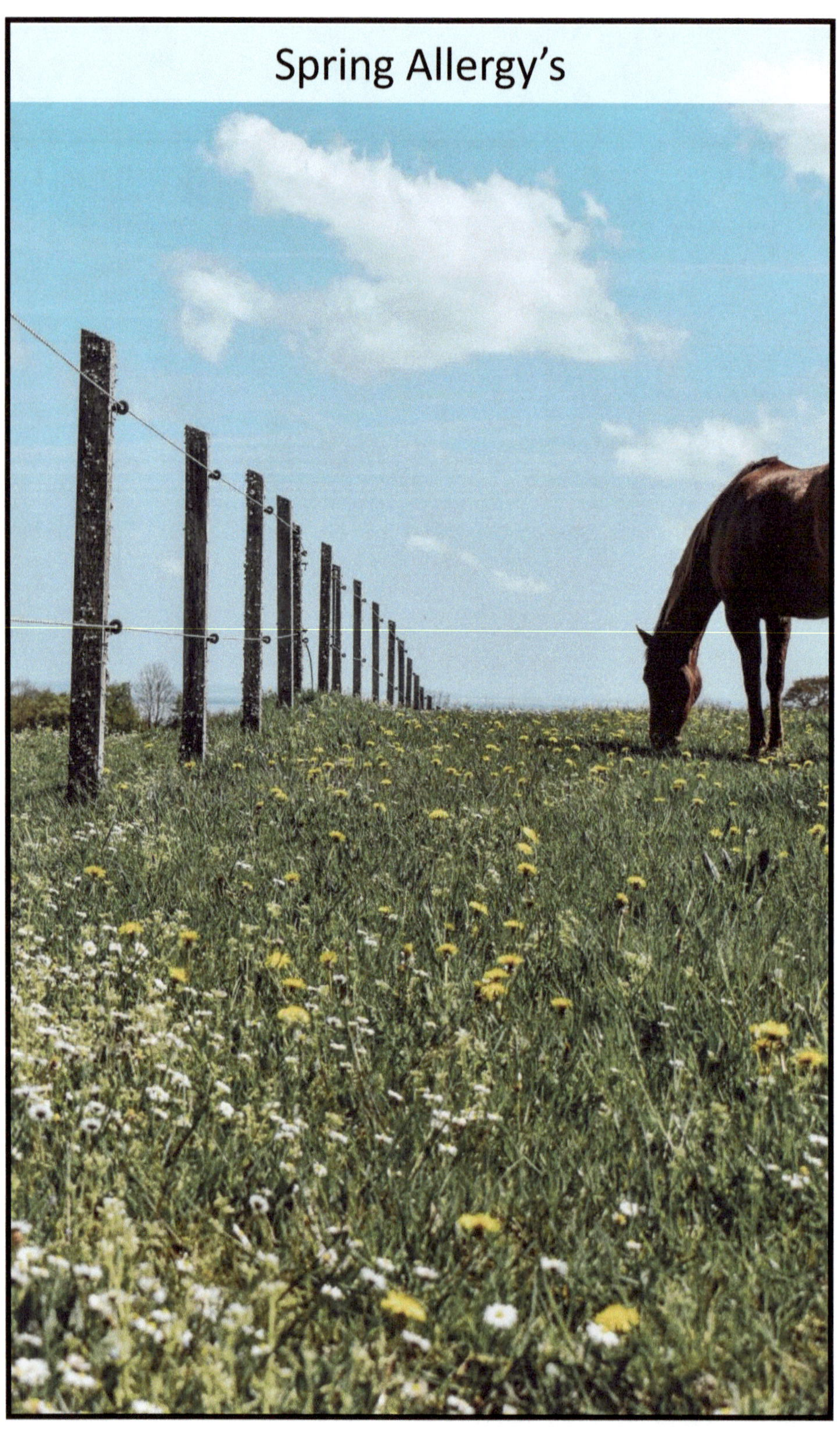